The Safe Food Handbook

THE EXPERIMENT

BECAUSE EVERY BOOK IS A TEST OF NEW IDEAS

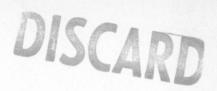

THE SAFE FOOD HANDBOOK

THE Safe Food HANDBOOK

HOW TO MAKE SMART CHOICES ABOUT RISKY FOOD

HELI PERRETT, PhD

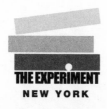

THE EXPERIMENT

NEW YORK

The Experiment, LLC
260 Fifth Avenue
New York, NY 10001-6425
www.theexperimentpublishing.com

Many of the designations used by manufacturers and sellers to distinguish their products are claimed as trademarks. Where those designations appear in this book and The Experiment was aware of a trademark claim, the designations have been capitalized.

The Experiment's books are available at special discounts when purchased in bulk for premiums and sales promotions as well as for fundraising or educational use. For details, contact us at info@theexperimentpublishing.com.

Note to Readers: This book contains food safety information and advice based on currently available information and best practice. Neither the author nor the publisher is engaged in rendering professional medical or other advice or services to individual readers, and accepts no liability or responsibility for possible injury resulting from any information herein or suggestion made. If you believe you have ingested contaminated food, contact your doctor or call 911. You may also want to consult the emergency numbers listed in Appendix 3 (Getting Help, page 312). The opinions expressed in this book represent the personal views of the author and not of the publisher.

Library of Congress Control Number: 2009940035

ISBN 978-1-61519-017-1

Cover design by Howard Grossman | 12E Design
Cover photographs © Fotolia.com
Text design by Pauline Neuwirth, Neuwirth & Associates, Inc.

Manufactured in the United States of America
First published January 2011
Published simultaneously in Canada

10 9 8 7 6 5 4 3 2 1

TO THOSE I DINE WITH.

Contents

Preface

T HE OTHER DAY, a friend asked me why I was writing this book. I answered, "I wrote it for you." She had just finished chemotherapy and had been told she had a weakened immune system, making her more vulnerable to infection and illness. At least two of my other friends were in similar situations. If, like them, you are in a high food-risk group because of illness or age, pregnancy, or medications you are taking, or have young children or other family members who are, I wrote it also for you.

Ultimately, if we value our health and want to live a long, active life, we *all* need to avoid contaminants and toxic substances in our food. Apart from anything else, no matter how delicious a meal may be—and I love food—food-borne illness is no fun. I am the poster child for what we venomously call "food poisoning": At least three serious incidents of bacteria-caused food-borne illness (one of which came close to costing me my life), three confirmed cases (probably four) of internal parasites . . . and who knows how many viruses, mold toxins, chemical toxins, and more. I don't need any proof that food can be risky.

There was the time I ate that delicious raw shellfish ceviche because I didn't want to offend the friend who was insisting I try it. Another time was when I was starving, late for a meeting, and I grabbed a Caesar salad (because it was quickest) at a restaurant I knew was unsanitary (I sat with my back to the open kitchen so that I couldn't see what was going on, which did not stop me from becoming ill). Another incident was probably caused by that undercooked barbecued chicken my husband made (he continues to deny it, but has since stopped barbecuing). And I am sure yet another experience involved slightly odd-smelling cold cuts in my refrigerator that were the only edible thing in the house when I returned late at night from a trip. One of the two worst times was when I ended up in intensive care with massive loss of blood. The other was when I became ill after working on sanitation in refugee camps in Bangladesh. (Believe me, it is very unpleasant to be violently ill on a long flight.) I have learned my lesson—but a little late. You could argue that it gives me an "inside view" of the issue. Frankly, I could have done without the personal experience.

It is not just a sudden bout of illness that we need to avoid. The subtle longer-term erosion of our health by toxic substances in our food may be even worse. I am fully convinced that hazards in our food are contributing to our constant fatigue and many of those debilitating and mysterious chronic conditions and diseases we suffer from—arthritis, digestive disorders, thyroid conditions, liver problems, cancers, and more. Why doesn't anyone laugh when I say that? Maybe deep down we all know it is true—but we don't want to think about it.

The pages that follow have drawn from thousands of sources and represent years of research on my part. Such sources cover a wide range: Statistics, original research, published books, scientific journal articles, case reports, expert committee reports (both in the North America and overseas), opinion pieces, government documents, and just about everything else relevant that I could lay my hands on. I also personally conducted limited interviews and observation studies, to check on issues. I have selected what I used with care, always going back to the original research whenever I could, and always using cross-verification with multiple different sources (through a process that the social sciences call **triangulation** [see note, page 1]) so that I would get the facts right. I have tried to be balanced and fair—and no doubt sometimes failed.

Writing this book has been an oddly personal experience. Frequently, I have swung back and forth in time and between my wide-ranging professional and personal experiences. I recalled being a seven-year-old child, living on a small farm, tending chickens, milking cattle, harvesting vegetables. At other times I was sitting in the laboratory, staring amazed at how those bacteria on the petri dish were no longer proving to be susceptible to the usual **antibiotics**. Or I was gazing through a microscope, looking at parasites that you would never have expected to turn up in North America, or researching incredible and rather beautiful fungi (molds). Still at other times, I was wandering around third-world countries, working with farmers—as the so-called foreign expert. Usually (to my shame), I was on the side of conventional agriculture, promoting use of factory-style farming, chemical fertilizer, and pesticides, often under the auspices of international organizations. At other times I was working with communities or women on the sanitation-, health-, and food-related issues that affected them.

Writing the book itself has been punctuated with tending my urban backyard garden in California—currently standing at thirteen fruit trees, grape and berry vines, nine different vegetables, eight fresh herbs, and two emerging fishponds, in which I swear that one day I will raise our dinner (once I solve the problem of gulls and raccoons). There are no chickens at present, which is maybe just as well, considering zoning laws. But every once in a while, I keep threatening to get some again, when I want to unnerve my family.

It has all come together, in a way . . . the various strands of my professional and personal experience. In that sense, everything in these pages is not just scientific, but also subjective. Perhaps, above all, it springs from my love of food in general—not just growing it, but cooking it, presenting it, sharing it with family and friends—and best of all, eating it. For me, food is a visual as well as a culinary art—one that has to appeal to all the senses at once. That is why I so resent the fact that food can also carry risks—and why I confess that I sometimes cheat on my own advice. Life is a compromise.

In this book I wanted to take a food-focused view of the food-safety topic, not the usual perspective. I also wanted to touch on a few of our unfounded food fears, as well as the more real immediate and longer-term risks that we face.

Not everyone will agree with my conclusions or the decisions or actions proposed. There is so much disagreement in this field that it would be surprising if everybody did agree. The situation itself is constantly changing as our global and industrialized food system changes, emerging risks are discovered, and new studies are done.

I would like this book to do two things for you. First, I want to make you think more about what you eat. Second, I would like to help you eat more safely—if you want to. Not everyone is going to be like my agent, who after reading the book became a **community-supported agriculture** (CSA) member. But this handbook may convince you to take the food safety issue a bit more seriously, particularly if you are in a high-risk group.

—Heli Perrett
Oakland, California

| **1** |

Check Your
Food-Risk Rating

W<small>E ALL WANT</small> to be healthy. What we eat is important to how we feel and how long we live. The nutritional value of our food is one important aspect. The food's safety is another. The more we can avoid illness-causing organisms, **toxic**[1] chemicals, and such other dangerous substances in our breakfast, lunch, and dinner, the better it is for us.

Can't we just eat the most nutritious food? Unfortunately, food safety and nutrition do not always agree. The "healthiest" fruits and vegetables, grains, and fish are not always the safest from **microbes** or from drug or **pesticide** residues. In fact, at times it can become a trade-off between nutrients and the safety of what we eat. Nor can we just rely on eating **organic, locally produced**, or **sustainably produced** food. Yes, often they are a better choice. But not always. Nor will buying the most expensive item give us any safety guarantees. In

---

1 Terms that appear in **boldface** on first use in the text are defined in the glossary, which begins on page 296.

fact, in some cases it can be the reverse: Many upmarket food retailers, which pride themselves on the wholesomeness of what they sell, issue constant product **recalls** because of contamination. There are also times that we can make an inexpensive type of food just as safe as the expensive one—if we know how to.

The large majority of **food hazards** are in our foods before we buy them. They have probably entered at the farm, the slaughter-house, the warehouse, the truck, or the retailer. It has been esti-mated that maybe four-fifths of food **contaminants** enter at the farm, or soon afterward, and the final fifth enter during process-ing. Smart purchasing decisions will help us choose the least **risky** foods available. In our own kitchens, we can either increase the risks that are already there, or reduce any existing risks—if we know how to.

Spoiled food is not always the same as unsafe food. "Bad food" may have started out safe, and often looks and smells the same as it always does. The riskiest food could be the one you least expect. Will it be your salad? your shrimp dish? your sushi? your French fries? your rice bran? your peanut snack? your hamburger? your tuna sandwich? The food that is riskiest today is often different from the one that was unsafe fifty years ago, two years ago—or even yester-day. So you can't always rely on what your mother told you. Or on that book you read ten years ago. Food risk is a moving target.

Naturally, the government tells us that our food is safe. What else could it say? In the United States, the statement is usually carefully phrased along the lines of: "The American food supply is *one of the safest* in the world" or "Our food supply continues to be *among the safest* in the world." But it is estimated that one in four Americans become ill from their food every year—perhaps closer to one in two, if you count all those misdiagnosed and unreported cases and all those milder cases for which we never see a doctor. The situation in Canada is similar.

Food-borne illness, a.k.a. food poisoning, is only the tip of the iceberg. It is now recognized that around 2 percent of victims of short bouts may end up with chronic health conditions. Research is looking into links between certain types of food-borne illness and those common diseases and health conditions many of us suffer from at some point in our life, ones such as arthritis, thyroid problems, inflammatory bowel disease, Crohn's disease, rheumatic heart disease, multiple sclerosis, kidney problems, and diabetes.

SALMONELLA EVERYWHERE

Salmonella infection (properly known as salmonellosis) is one of our most common food-borne illnesses. It seems that every time we turn around, *Salmonella* **bacteria** are there, contaminating one of our foods—our leafy greens, our tomatoes, our peppers, our meat, our eggs, our dairy, our baked goods, our peanuts and tree nuts, and even our spices. Remember the nationwide recall of half a billion shell eggs in August 2010? That was caused by *Salmonella* bacteria. What is happening?

There are a number of reasons that this is turning into such a problem. One is that we are not just seeing one kind of *Salmonella* but several subspecies and thousands of **serovars** (strains), many of which can make us ill. In fact, they have probably been causing illness for thousands of years. Two strains, *Salmonella enteritidis* and *Salmonella typhimurium,* are the most common in the United States and account for half of all *Salmonella* infections in humans. Another reason we are seeing so many of them in our food is that *Salmonella* bacteria are everywhere in nature (in soil, water, plants, and animals) as well as in many of our food-processing plants. So it would be surprising if they did *not* get into our food. *Salmonella* travels around—from animals to the soil, from soil to plants, from plants back to animals.

Another reason that *Salmonella* bacteria turn up so often is that these bacteria are very hardy. They have been known to survive for years in soil and for months in dry places where one wouldn't expect them to. In fact, salmonellosis **outbreaks** have been linked to a number of fairly dry food products, such as chocolate, powdered milk, black pepper, and desiccated coconut. Even living in pepper, they still multiply. Foods that are contaminated with *Salmonella* usually look, smell, and taste normal.

It is believed that *Salmonella* could be causing as many as 1.3 million illnesses every year in the United States. Although *Salmonella* bacteria are usually not quite as vicious as some *E. coli* strains, such as *E. coli* O147 and O145, they can be pretty dangerous—to some people. Symptoms of *Salmonella* infection are typical of food poisoning. They will usually develop twelve to seventy-two hours after eating contaminated food. Healthy people may just have four to seven days of **diarrhea**, nausea, vomiting, and abdominal cramps—and may lose as much as ten pounds. Many recover with no treatment at all. But for young children, the elderly, and people with a weakened **immune system**, an infection by *Salmonella* can be very serious: The bacteria can invade the bloodstream and infect other parts of their body, such as their heart, kidneys, liver, or brain. Some studies argue that people over age fifty-five seem to be most seriously affected by *Salmonella*, and end up in the hospital.

What most people are not aware of is, once their bout with salmonellosis appears to be over, it may not be over. For a small percentage of individuals (much higher among those who have had a serious episode), there can be longer-term health complications. Also, some people who recover from a salmonella infection can also become carriers of the bacteria, without any symptoms. If they are food-service workers and are not scrupulously sanitary in their practices, they could contribute to all those salmonellosis outbreaks.

On top of all the cases of "food poisoning" that grab the headlines, we also have an unseen longer-term accumulation of food-associated risks—occurring without any sudden bout of illness involved. These risks tend to be related to devious agricultural and industrial pollutants that add to our **body burden** of toxic substances, meal after meal. It could be that those tiny regular **doses** of toxic substances, such as certain pesticides, dioxins, **PCBs**, arsenic, and **mercury**, are contributing to many of our worst diseases and most mysterious syndromes, including cancer, Alzheimer's, fibromyalgia, **ADHD** (attention-deficit/hyperactivity disorder—see sidebar), autism, Asperger's syndrome, Reye's syndrome, and many others. Some studies and experts argue that there is a link. Others disagree. We don't have final answers yet. What we do know is that Americans—and a large number of American children—have the world's highest body burden of some of these toxic substances.

ARE PESTICIDES CONTRIBUTING TO ADHD?

ADHD is a common medical condition that may affect as many as one in twenty children in the United States, and many adults. Symptoms of ADHD include hyperactivity, inattention, and impulsivity. The disorder has enormous social and economic costs to families and society.

We are still not quite sure what causes ADHD. Ongoing research is looking into genetic causes; abnormal brain development; allergies; premature birth; the mother's use of cigarettes, alcohol or drugs; lead exposure; and sugar and food additives in the diet of the children themselves. Now there is new evidence that pesticides may also be playing a role.

A research study reported in the *Journal of the American Academy of Pediatrics* (May 17, 2010), found a positive association between body levels of organophosphates—a general name for insecticides commonly used on fruits and vegetables—and ADHD in American children ages eight to fifteen. This was a well-done and reasonably large and representative study, carried out by leading U.S. and Canadian universities. The levels of organophosphates used in the research are quite common among American children. The study concluded that organophosphates may be contributing to ADHD prevalence.

Who is at most risk? "Bad food" does not affect everyone equally. If you are a healthy adult, well armed with an immune system, **gastrointestinal** tract, liver, and kidneys that are all functioning optimally, your body will be better able to deal with invaders of all kinds. But some people are very vulnerable. A family of four can eat the same contaminated chicken and salad dinner with quite different results. One person may feel just a little "off" and tired for a couple of days, another may come down with moderate gastrointestinal symptoms, and two may end up in the hospital. Also, with certain food hazards, if you just take antacids, or a certain antibiotic, or have a couple of glasses of wine with dinner, your vulnerability can increase substantially. But usually higher risk is linked to life stage, health, and diet. See "Are You in a High-Risk Group?" to see whether either you, or a member of your family, fall or might fall into a high food-risk category, either now or in the future.

ARE YOU IN A HIGH-RISK GROUP?

People that are most likely to be affected by risky foods usually fall into four main groups, largely based on age and health.

◇ **Infants and young children**—because their body and brain are still developing and because they eat a limited range of foods, thus concentrating their risk. In the case of certain toxic substances, they are also likely to pick up larger additional doses from the environment than are adults.

◇ **Pregnant women**—who are at greater risk of developing certain food-borne illnesses and whose unborn child is also at risk. Some toxic substances that accumulate in the body can also be passed through breast milk by nursing mothers.

◇ **People with weakened immune systems or chronic health conditions**—as in the case of those who have diabetes, cancer, HIV/AIDS, or another serious illness or condition such as abnormal liver or kidney function or weakened digestive processes. This category also includes those who are taking certain over-the-counter or prescription medications, such as steroids; certain medications to fight autoimmune disease; and drugs given after organ transplant, which can reduce the ability to fight disease.

◇ **Elderly people**—because as we age, our body's ability to deal with toxic organisms and substances decreases. Even a mild food-borne illness can have fatal consequences.

If you look at the high-risk groups, you will realize that we all normally fall into at least two of them at some time in our lifetime. Even if you are not currently in a high-risk group, the chances are that you care about someone who is—such as a child, or an ill or elderly relative or partner.

Perhaps I should also mention the obvious issue—diet. Some types of diets are riskier than others, for a variety of reasons. Review yours as you read this book. Note that your risk will be affected not only by what you usually eat, but by its diversity or lack thereof. One issue with many of us these days is habitually consuming just a few foods. If you eat mainly pizza, pasta, and burgers, you are consuming primarily wheat, cheese, tomatoes, and ground meat, and will therefore be more than normally affected by anything toxic in these food items. The same would apply if you dine at the other end of the spectrum, following a raw-food diet. In that case, you may be more vulnerable to common contaminants in raw fruits and vegetables and nuts than is someone who eats a wider variety of foods and eats them cooked. Again, if you have salmon for breakfast every day, and spinach salads just about every night for dinner—as a friend of mine does—your diet may not actually be the safest. My point is, lack of diversity concentrates your risk. It's rather like investing all your money in General Motors, Citibank, and Microsoft. Even though the stocks are in different sectors, they are still just three companies. If General Motors goes under—you may, too.

2

What Makes Our Food Risky?

Not everything we eat is equally risky. Some foods and places to eat are more likely to be so than others. But, given the right circumstances, any food can be hazardous to our health—not just our leafy greens or seafood or meat, but even (sadly) our chocolate, soft drinks, and yogurt. Who would have thought that peanuts would be one of our most frightening foods? In recent years there have been incidents of various forms of contamination in such unexpected food items as dry cereal, children's candy, peanut butter, ice pops, popcorn, "pure" bottled water, coffee, pepper, and superhealthy drink mixes.

Four Kinds of Food Hazards

Food hazards vary as well. We tend to think of them in terms of bacteria, such as *E. coli* O157:H7 and *Salmonella,* and maybe pesticide residues. We are learning that bacteria are the ultimate survivors—and ruthless opportunists. But there are many other risks. Most, but not all, of the dangers you need to watch for in your food fall into four groups:

- **Microorganisms and the toxins they produce:** Microbes such as bacteria, **viruses, parasites,** or **fungi (molds),** can enter our food at any stage between farm and table—in the field, a waterway, in a barn or slaughterhouse; during storage, processing, packing, or transport; at our favorite restaurant or neighborhood store; or inside our own kitchen. All it takes is a little contaminated soil or irrigation water or one tiny slip-up by a farm, warehouse, or food-service worker—or by you or me. It has been estimated that close to half of our raw food is likely to contain small numbers of some dangerous microorganism or other, many of which we have never heard of. Some estimates put it closer to 100 percent. Unluckily for us, those millions of different kinds of microbes are everywhere— in the soil, water, air, on our face and hands, and on our kitchen counter. Some are harmless, but some are very dangerous to our health.

- **Toxic industrial and agricultural chemicals:** Toxic chemicals are everywhere as well, and it is very difficult to keep them out of our food. Today's farmers and industry are not to blame for many of the worst of these. The group called persistent organic pollutants (**POPs**) are among the most toxic compounds ever made. They include ones like **DDT,** aldrin, **dieldrin,** chlordane, toxaphene, PCBs, hexachlorobenzene, and unintentionally produced toxic wastes such as dioxins and furans. Many POPs are still around, in spite of bans and environmental cleanup attempts, and keep turning up in our food and animal feed—which passes along to our meat and milk and farmed fish. Studies show that we are "eating POPs" in foods such as farmed fish, fatty meat and chicken, and whole-milk dairy foods (see page 14). In addition, we have all those new pollutants that are constantly being produced—plus some naturally occurring metals that can be toxic if we are exposed to too much of them.

- **Drugs and hormones:** These are given to many of our food animals and our increasingly popular farmed fish. Industrial farming practices have a lot to do with it. Frequently the immediate reason for veterinary drug use is for preventing—not curing—disease, and for enhancing productivity or growth—and profits. Governments and scientists are increasingly concerned that such use of antibiotics is contributing to development of **superbugs**—those multidrug-resistant bacteria that we all fear. Such bacteria are already turning up in our imported shrimp and in our meat. Although the use of hormones still remains a controversial issue, there are enough unpleasant research findings about them to worry those concerned with food safety.
- **Natural toxins:** Under certain conditions, some shellfish and plants can produce compounds that are toxic to humans if ingested, or ingested in sufficient quantities. (So can some herbal supplements—not discussed in this book.) Just because they are natural does not make them any better for us than industrial or agricultural toxins. In fact, some of these natural chemicals are among the most fast-acting and toxic substances we can find in our food. They are often impossible to destroy, their effects are hard for our doctors to diagnose, and they are frequently difficult to deal with once they are in our bodies.

All these four kinds of contaminants *exist* in our foods. It is not a question of *whether* they are there, but *how much* is there. But aren't they controlled for by established tolerance levels and monitoring of our food supply? Well, yes and no.

Action levels and tolerances (meaning levels above which the government will take legal action) have been established for many of the most dangerous organisms and poisonous substances in our food and are being regularly monitored. For instance, the level of the potent mold toxin **aflatoxin** allowed in your child's milk is 0.5 ppb, but is 20 ppb in peanut butter. Your potatoes, carrots, beets, and horseradish are allowed to carry up to 0.1 ppb of toxic aldrin or dieldrin, or of chlordane. Those same carrots can also hold as much as 3.0 ppb of DDT and your fish as much as 5.0 ppb before the U.S. Food and Drug Administration (FDA) steps in. Even red meat can have as much as 5 ppb of nasty PCBs before action is taken.

But of the huge number of contaminants that could turn up in our North American food supply, only a minuscule fraction have been thoroughly studied and are being checked (see page 42). Remember the *E. coli* O145 bacteria that were found in shredded romaine lettuce in 2010, when we were just focusing on *E. coli* O147:H7? And do you recall the 2008 case of Mexico's rejecting a large shipment of U.S. beef because their testing turned up copper levels that exceeded those considered safe for human consumption in Mexico? It has been rumored that U.S diners ended up eating that beef—perfectly legally. Why? Because the United States government didn't have any tolerance levels for copper in beef.

Again, as you will see in the pages that follow, the North American action levels and tolerances are often set higher than those of the European Union (EU) and other countries. Are we really supposed to be tougher? This makes me uncomfortable. So does the fact that different nations, scientists, and even our own government agencies do not always agree on how much is too much of one toxic risk or another. They also change their mind on a fairly regular basis. A substance declared perfectly safe for the last twenty years could be considered unsafe tomorrow.

Other factors affect how safe our foods may be. Testing (and taking a sample) to check on toxic levels in food is often not 100 percent reliable. In addition, many of us are exposed to toxic substances from several sources, say, from a couple of the foods we eat and our drinking water, plus from our bedroom carpet and our lawn spray. This adds up. Or we may be getting more than usual because of lack of diversity in our diet. Or we may be particularly vulnerable to their effect, to start off with. And what about synergistic effects of one of these substances with another, which hardly anybody seems to be looking at?

Why Isn't Our Food Becoming Safer?

FOOD-BORNE ILLNESS is not new. Nor are toxic chemicals and metals in food. Nor are attempts to make food safer to eat. The Greek botanist Theophrastus (370–285 BCE), the Roman Pliny the Elder (23–79 CE), and the ancient Greek physician Galen (129–199 CE) were concerned about food safety, even though they knew nothing about bacteria or some of the other risks we worry about today. Efforts to regulate the safety of what people eat date back at least to Roman civil law. The U.S. federal framework for food safety—which survives today—is based on the Pure Food and Drug Act of 1906. In Canada, the first federal legislation dealing with safety of food (and drink) was enacted as early as 1874. The current legislative framework for food safety was established by the Food and Drugs Act first passed in 1920 and later revised.

We would expect that with all the advances in science, technology, and safety procedures, our food has become incrementally safer over the years. Instead, the data show that we are not meeting our goals of reducing food-borne illness, or of reducing levels of some of those toxic chemicals. Yes, this is the case in spite of special targeted programs and efforts. Some food hazards even show signs of becoming worse, such as veterinary drugs in food. Whatever improvements *are* made are not able to keep up with changes in the way our food is produced and distributed, and the way that food risks, themselves, are changing.

To set the scene for the more micro-focused and practical chapters that follow, let's take a quick look at some of the factors that are helping to keep our food unsafe.

. . .

Our food system is becoming more and more complex and industrialized. This factor multiplies any problems that occur, with larger numbers and wider geographic spread of victims, and often slow response to outbreaks.

Feeding North America has become a massive, complex, globalized, and highly industrialized operation, involving hundreds of thousands of producers, distributors, transporters, and processors, some of these in-country and others overseas. How can any food safety agency regularly check on all these actors to make sure they are obeying the safety regulations?

The food industry is dominated by a relatively small number of large and powerful companies. These own or control production inputs such as seed, fertilizer, land, and livestock; the production and harvesting processes; and the processing, packaging, and distribution of food products. They employ factory-style, assembly-line operations; use large amounts of land, water, **synthetic fertilizers**, pesticides, hormones, and antibiotics; and carry out massive harvesting and slaughter operations. Forget your image of the red-cheeked smiling farmer standing in front of a picture-perfect red barn and happily grazing cows, who sells what he produces to the local store. He—or she—is an endangered species.

The bulk of our food moves through many stages and travels over thousands of miles before it reaches our plate. A single finished food item can source ingredients from suppliers all over the country and from overseas and ship its finished products nationwide under a wide variety of brand names. Two halves of a pecan nut, from the same Georgia grower, can turn up under several different product names. Lettuce or spinach leaves from the same Salinas, California, lettuce plant can end up being sold in both bagged and loose forms, mixed and unmixed with other leafy greens, in many parts of the country.

Product mixing is one of the riskier aspects of this modern food supply. Tomatoes, berries, grains, nuts, and other products from different farms—and sometimes from different countries—are frequently mixed together. Days and even months of storage in warehouses and time on the road allows microbial contaminations to spread, encourages the use of fumigants to avoid them, and makes back-tracing difficult when outbreaks occur.

The food-growing environment is still contaminated. Even if some of the worst chemical threats, such as those POPs mentioned earlier, are slowly being reduced, more and more toxic compounds are finding their way into our soil, water, and air. They result from activities in industry, energy, mining, and other aspects of modern life, such as traffic and golf-course maintenance. From there they can enter our water supply and our food. Pesticides used in agriculture are, of course, another source. The Center for Disease Control and Prevention (CDC) estimates that more than a billion pounds of pesticide-active ingredients are used each year in the United States, mostly, but not entirely, by farmers. More than sixteen thousand pesticide products are being marketed in America. Who knows what all these pesticides are? Only time will *really* tell what these substances are doing to our food and our body. Some of them do not even have to be registered, if they manage to qualify as "minimum-risk pesticides." Some don't have to have any established "maximum residue levels" or be monitored if they manage to qualify for the Environmental Protection Agency (EPA) exemption. Who has the time (or money) to test them all, let alone for any longer-term effects on our health?

And POPs that may have been used years ago, or far away, are still around, too, in a kind of half-life. "Nowhere to Hide," a 2000 study by the Pesticide Action Network of North America (PANNA), although somewhat dated now, found that a holiday dinner menu with eleven food items could give the diner thirty-eight "POP hits" (a *hit* being defined as one persistent toxic chemical on one food item). Other more recent studies have also confirmed continuing POP presence in our foods and in cattle and fish feed (and from there, are entering our food). Several can even be carried for miles by air currents and storm systems (and easily across the fence to my organic vegetables if my neighbor sprays his blackberry vines). Research has also found that, in spite of bans, several of the most toxic chemicals are still being used by some of the countries from which we import our food these days. Crops such as root and leafy vegetables can pick them up from the soil. Cattle and fish eat them in their feed. When POPs are in our food, we ingest them. Even mothers' milk can be contaminated with such toxins if the mother has been exposed. That is why the government establishes those action levels—because it acknowledges that such poisonous substances in our food are "unavoidable" (that is the exact word the FDA uses).

These toxic compounds can build up in our body over time, mouthful by mouthful and milligram by milligram.

More and more of our food is imported from overseas. Yes, all those imports give us wonderful choices. But we pay for our globalized food with more risks in the food we eat.

We import tens of billions of dollars of food (and drink) annually. The United States imports food from more than 150 nations. More of this imported food is coming from developing nations or newly industrialized countries. Frequently they have risky production, harvesting, transport, storage, and processing practices; highly contaminated soil, air and waterways; and unreliable electricity and road conditions. In theory, all imported food products have to meet the same safety standards as domestically produced foods. But this is difficult to assure. Yes, there *are* food safety standards and guidelines for overseas producers, distributors, and processors. But often they are poorly enforced and easily circumvented.

Some research suggests that imported foods may be as many as three times more likely to expose us to dangerous pesticide residues, and more likely to carry **pathogenic** bacteria and parasites and drug residues. Other research says, "It depends." Of course, the degree of risk does vary with the country, the particular overseas producer or plant, and so many other factors. If you look at the percentage of incoming shipments that are approved (that is, not rejected) by inspectors, clearly imports of food from Canada to the United States, and from the United States to Canada, have a much better track record than those from most other countries such as India, China, Mexico, and Vietnam.

Our government's ability to inspect overseas food facilities or inspect incoming shipments is very limited. On those relatively few occasions when overseas plant inspections are scheduled, the local government's regulations can prevent access to our inspectors, and logistics, cultural, and language differences can create roadblocks to getting an accurate picture of the situation. I have seen these problems and know how real they are. Food safety, as we in North America understand it, does not have the same priority with some of our trading partners, and value systems and attitudes toward regulations are different.

In theory, incoming food products are inspected at our borders. But in practice, the large majority of the millions of products that enter our ports every year and end up on our dinner plate are *uninspected* and untested on arrival. The resources to examine every shipment are just not available. The number of incoming products has multiplied in recent years, and safety agency budgets have lagged far behind. So, how much of imported food *is* inspected? In the United States, probably somewhere between 0.7 to 1.5 percent of shipments coming in through the more than three hundred ports, with some variation between different food products (for instance, more inspection of shellfish and meat than of fruit). Let's say it is a little more than 1 percent. That means we just have to hope for the best for the remaining 99 percent or so of the imported foods we eat.

China is now one of the most important sources of food imports for the United States (see sidebar). Between 2001 and 2008, U.S. food imports from China more than tripled in value, reaching $5.2 billion. Only Mexico and Canada are more important. But China appears to be increasing its import share, particularly as the supplier of some of our riskiest foods, such as farmed seafood and ready-to-eat products.

U.S. IMPORTED FOOD FROM CHINA—A GROWING CONCERN

China exports an enormous variety of agriculture and seafood products to the United States—more than 40 percent of our fish and seafood (mainly farmed), 10 percent of our shrimp, about 50 percent of our garlic, more than 60 percent of our apple juice, and a large proportion of our canned, pickled, and dried fruit, vegetables, and nut products. Fish and shellfish are not only the largest but also the fastest-growing category.

In recent years there has been growing concern within safety agencies, in U.S. Congress, and among consumers, about the safety of Chinese imports in general, from children's toys to all-terrain vehicles (ATVs) to drywall to shrimp. Many of the food-related concerns are based on China's growing environmental pollution, its heavy use of agricultural chemicals and veterinary drugs, its poor food handling and storage practices (some due to power outages), and its generally weak enforcement of food safety standards. The 2008 **melamine**-adulterated milk powder (in which hundreds of thousands of infants were sickened in China itself) and the melamine pet food contamination incident in North America (which caused the death by kidney failure of untold numbers of cats and dogs) have added to such concerns.

Some analyses of rejected shipments have found double, or even greater frequency, of import rejects from China than from other countries. A review of the Food and Drug Administration (FDA)'s recent inspections of incoming food imports from China shows a constant array of positive checks for such categories as "filth" (insects, human hair, feces, dirt), illegal **food additives** such as colorings, **carcinogenic** drug residues, mold, and *Salmonella* bacteria.

We have underestimated the survival powers of food hazards. This applies not only to POPs, which we already mentioned, but to microbes. Microorganisms—bacteria, molds, viruses, parasites—remain a constant threat in our food. Many of our past assumptions about the vulnerability of bacteria and other microbes are turning out to be wrong, or at best partially true.

As discussed on page 272, some bacteria, for example, certain species of *Salmonella*, can survive in dried spices such as paprika and chili powder for months. *Listeria monocytogenes* can multiply in our cooler or refrigerator while hiding in our hot dogs or cold cuts and survive in the freezer. We used to think that contaminants lurking on the outside of fruit, vegetables, eggs, and nuts could be washed away. We now know that they can also burrow their way right through the peel or shell. We also used to think that thorough cooking would kill anything; we are now finding out that certain microbes can survive high heat or perish yet leave their toxins behind.

Antibiotics used to be a great solution for curing any bacteria-caused illness we had. We are now discovering that an increasing number of bacteria are no longer susceptible to our most popular and powerful drugs. Without adequate financial incentives, new and more effective drugs are not being produced fast enough to take their place. Similarly, we used to think of mold toxins as simply something we didn't want in our house. Now they are turning up in many of our foods. And, although we didn't think much about norovirus as a food contaminant because it does not make us as ill as some other microbes, it has begun cropping up too frequently in places we are meant to be enjoying ourselves—such as weddings and cruise ships—and in school lunches. If that isn't enough, parasites may be making a steady comeback, helped along by globalization of our food supply, the number of "carrier" food-service workers, and our own travel.

Our Own Choices Help to Increase Risks

IT IS EASIER TO put the blame for unsafe food onto the big players—the food industry or government—than to blame ourselves. True, to some extent, we consumers are at their mercy.

Recent outbreaks in our food supply have shown us that neither is doing very well in protecting us. But let's be fair: We are not guilt-free, either. Our eating preferences are playing a role in making our meals less safe.

Global eating is adding to our risks. We already mentioned our increasing food imports. But we have to remember that our own eating preferences are playing a part in this. In the old days, we used to eat what was available locally and in season, without a great deal of variety. These days, we want our favorite foods when we want them—all the time. Oddly enough, several consumer surveys I have looked at say that the large majority of us don't really *trust* imported food. But that doesn't mean we don't eat it. Americans are now believed to be eating somewhere between 260 and 300 pounds of imported food per person per year (estimates vary). The amount has almost doubled since the mid-1990s. Although there is some fluctuation month to month and year to year, the U.S. Department of Agriculture (USDA) estimates that imported food in the average American's diet amounts to about 30 percent of fruit, juices, and nuts; 10 percent of red meats; and close to 80 percent of fish and shellfish. Sitting at our table at home and eating just one prepared food can end up being an international experience. An item such as Chicken Cordon Bleu (made primarily of chicken, ham, cheese, and bread crumbs) may contain ingredients from ten different nations. Even the all-American hamburger can be global.

Our increasing love of imported foods has given us the variety and availability we like but has also put us at greater risk.

We are eating more ready and risky food. Let's face it—we are in love with convenience. As more of us work outside the home, we like to cook fast and eat fast, and we don't like to clean up a kitchen mess afterward. The process of cooking and eating can frequently become a race to the end—so that we can get on with something else. If we are honest, most of us will admit that rather than cook, we prefer to read a book about food, watch a cooking show on television, or surf recipes on the Internet (I love doing this, although, preferring to be "creative," I very rarely use a recipe). Besides, we can put our feet up while doing it.

No wonder ready-to-eat (RTE) foods have caught on so fast. So have ready-to-cook products such as pecan- and hazelnut-flavored salmon fillets (with a slice of lemon even provided) and the rosemary-and-garlic rubbed roast. RTE foods are great for our busy modern lifestyle. RTE food products cover a wide range, but are essentially those that one can eat without wasting time on washing or cooking or other forms of preparation. RTE foods include deli meats and poultry, sushi, sandwiches, and salads, as well as all those neat little plastic plates, trays, and containers of prewashed, sliced up, and artistically arranged helpings of fresh apple, cantaloupe, pineapple, celery, or carrots. More and more of these RTE foods are now imported. During the last decade, they have experienced more import growth than any other food category.

So what is wrong with a little convenience? Personally, as someone who is chronically rushed and always multitasking, I love to save time. Unfortunately, when it comes to food, ready = risky. There are several reasons. When "wounded" or cut up, certain foods, such as fruits and vegetables, are also more open to entry of bacteria or mold spores or viruses (see page 36). Outbreak statistics prove the point (see page 37). And we already mentioned the risks of mixing, which also applies to mixing different *kinds* of foods. *Salmonella* bacteria in a salad leaf can travel to the deli meat or the slice of cheese on your prepackaged sandwich and thrive even better.

Another reason why RTE foods are riskier is that they have gone through more stages than "simple" foods, and been handled by more people. This allows plenty of opportunities for contamination by food workers who are asymptomatic—or even symptomatic—carriers (remember Typhoid Mary?) who work while ill (quite common when workers are not paid for sick days). Surveys of those handling RTE foods have come up with some horrifying findings, suggesting that more than half may not wear gloves while preparing RTE foods, as required by health department regulations, and roughly a third do not wash their hands or change gloves or utensils between handling raw meat and an RTE food item. Almost a third of such workers may be carrying the dangerous *Listeria* or *Salmonella* bacteria in their gastrointestinal tract, and an estimated 25 to 30 percent are believed to be carrying *Staphylococcus aureus* bacteria [the one that can become the frightening antibiotic resistant MRSA (methicillin-resistant *Staphylococcus aureus*)] in their nose. How many hands actually touched your food? Were the utensils clean? Where was the food sitting during its preparation? How long and where was it stored, once it was ready?

Many of these "convenience" risks are discussed further later in this book. Convenience has a price, and not just what we pay at the checkout.

We love eating out and take-out. More frequent dining outside our homes is one of the great lifestyle changes of our age. It may cost us more, but it is also relaxing. Prior to the recession, studies showed that on the average, we either ate out or ordered take-out four to five times a week. Or even more, if we worked outside the home. The recession took its toll, apparently more so in the case of higher-end restaurants. Many of the usual eaters-out traded down or ended up getting take-out food. But this is changing as more people find jobs and incomes recover. Recent government estimates show that fifty cents of every U.S. food dollar is spent on food prepared outside our home (RTE foods, restaurant meals, or take-out).

From a safety point of view, eating out and take-out are much the same thing. Much as we love it, eating at restaurants or eating take-out food is normally riskier than eating food you cook at home— that is, unless you *really* don't know what you are doing. According to the CDC, about half of food-based illnesses originate in restaurants, which is more than the proportion of meals or food eaten there, and more than the number of food-related illnesses anywhere else. This is why some oncologists advise their cancer patients to avoid eating out until their immune systems recover. It is not just a matter of finding a bug, dead or alive, in our food, or glimpsing a cockroach or mouse scampering across the floor of the restaurant. There is a lot that we can't see that can make us sick.

Restaurant kitchen staff are usually part of the problem. Of course, restaurants have strict policies on sanitary practices such as hand-washing, often posted in two languages. But studies have shown that a frightening number of employees don't follow them. If you really want to be turned off eating out, read some of the restaurant worker blogs. And despite what you may think, expensive does not necessarily mean better.

An analysis of forty thousand New York Department of Health and Mental Hygiene restaurant inspection records for a typical month—February 2009—reveals that 34 percent of restaurants were found to have conditions that encouraged vermin, 29 percent had signs of rodents, 22 percent did not keep cold food at the proper temperature for safety, 17 percent did not protect food from contamination, and 19 percent had improper plumbing. These are just some of the noted problems. The performance of restaurants in other cities is not much better. Unfortunately, punishments for restaurants that violate sanitation standards are relatively mild. In worst cases, fees and penalties are handed out, but reinspection only occurs in a small percentage.

Partly, restaurants are riskier simply because they operate like restaurants (see sidebar).

WHY IS IT RISKIER TO EAT OUT THAN AT HOME?

Apart from any sanitation problems, safety risks are simply built into the way that restaurants operate.

◇ Restaurants tend to prepare foods in bulk. This can result in mixing together, or "pooling," items (such as eggs, one of which can be bad and contaminate the rest), and can make it more difficult to evenly control the temperature of the entire pot or batch when cooking and cooling.

◇ Often foods have to be prepared ahead of time, which allows dangerous bacteria and other microbes to get in and start reproducing before you order and eat the food.

◇ Food may not be stored at the right temperature, particularly in a busy restaurant, because of capacity problems, employee carelessness, or broken cooling or warming equipment.

◇ **Cross-contamination** can occur quite easily between raw and cooked foods because cutting boards, knives, and other food preparation tools are used multiple times, by different chefs, sometimes without washing in between.

◇ As restaurants face difficult times, slightly "off" foods may be served anyway, to increase profits.

◇ Many different people are involved in preparing meals, some of them poorly paid and trained, with chronic bacterial and parasite illnesses, often without adequate supervision.

Based on www.foodpoisoningprevention.com.

Why Aren't Government and the Food Industry Doing More?

GOVERNMENT AND THE food industry share responsibility for the safety of our food supply. The government provides a regulatory framework and guidance for the delivery of safe food, whereas the industry is responsible for making sure that the food it makes available to us is safe enough to eat. Both are making improvements, but not enough to keep up with the range and complexity of risks.

Government is having a hard time keeping up. The U.S. government's performance is hampered by lack of resources and the limits posed by outdated regulations, technology, and procedures. Its strategies and priorities are still largely based on the food supply and risks of the early twentieth century—not the twenty-first. The situation is made worse by the division of food safety responsibilities among some dozen federal agencies (depending on how you count), implementing some thirty different laws. The main federal government agencies responsible for both domestic and imported foods are the FDA (part of the U.S. Department of Health and Human Services), and the USDA's Food Safety and Inspection Service (USDA/FSIS). The FDA, and really just one small part of it—the Center for Food Safety and Applied Nutrition (CFSAN)—oversees about 80 percent of U.S. domestic and imported foods.

Examples of FDA-regulated foods include seafood, fruits and vegetables, dairy products, whole eggs, and most processed foods. The USDA is responsible for regulation of most of our meat and poultry and for egg products. Over the years, both the FDA and USDA have suffered from serious financial constraints. The FDA's budget increases haven't kept up. The food imports it has to regulate have tripled in just one decade. New responsibilities are being added regularly, and the agency's energies are being constantly diverted to food crisis management.

Other agencies playing a key role in the United States are the Centers for Disease Control and Prevention (CDC) and the Environmental Protection Agency (EPA). The CDC's responsibilities include investigating food-related illnesses and outbreaks and conducting surveillance of several food-borne pathogens and of control efforts. The EPA's Office of Prevention, Pesticides and Toxic Substances (OPTS) is in charge of protecting the environment from dangerous pesticides and toxic chemicals. It establishes those action levels and tolerances for toxic substances in our food that we talked about earlier. These are then enforced by the FDA and USDA.

The FDA and USDA/FSIS work with several hundred state agencies across the United States that do most of the actual inspections of foods and food facilities in their respective states. Ideally, this system promotes and enforces food safety regulations, links up with the food industry to make sure it is following safe practices, makes sure food is labeled correctly, educates consumers, and, when needed, tracks down the cause of outbreaks.

In Canada there is also shared responsibility for food safety, but the system is simpler and operates in a more centralized and integrated way. Health Canada (HC) is responsible for setting the policies and standards for both the nutritional quality and the safety of all food sold in Canada. The Canadian Food Inspection Agency (CFIA) enforces them. The CFIA conducts all *federal* food inspection activities, and also has responsibilities for animal health and plant protection. A very good aspect of the Canadian system is that the CFIA oversees the whole food continuum (before and after agricultural production). It collaborates with provincial and territorial health departments in carrying out its activities. Provincial governments regulate food retailers and services such as restaurants. Other Canadian agencies that play important roles are the Public Health Agency of Canada (PHAC) and, under CFIA guidance, the Canada Border Services Agency (CBSA), which is responsible for the initial import inspection of food.

The food industry's approach to safety is based on self-interest. This is not surprising because, after all, it is out to make a profit. This determines its attitude toward any safety measures. If there is a clear payoff in terms of preventing costly product recalls or winning back disillusioned consumers, it is likely to go along with stricter regulations or new measures. Recalls of contaminated products are the last thing it wants—with reason. They are very costly and risk harming the company image. (Maybe that is why so few company Web sites say anything about an ongoing recall of their products.) Although they are better than nothing, they don't always work best for us, either (see sidebar).

DON'T RELY ON FOOD RECALLS

A food recall is a measure of last resort—when it is too late to do anything else to protect consumers. In essence, the company responsible for a contaminated food product is also responsible for immediately informing the retailers or other companies that have received it, doing everything it can to get every single hazardous frozen hamburger or lettuce leaf or pistachio nut back, and making sure there is no way those items can ever enter the (human) food system again. It also has to make sure that the cause of the problem is fixed. The government's role is to keep an eye on the situation and to provide a push if needed. On rare occasions, it takes over the recall itself. This may be increasing under new legislation.

Many of us associate food risks with well-publicized recalls such as the 2010 nationwide shell egg *Salmonella* outbreak, which sickened at least 1,500 people, and the 2008-2009 peanut-product-linked outbreak that resulted in more than 650 illnesses and at least nine deaths in forty-five U.S. states and Canada. The latter led to recall of thousands of suspect food products, cost the peanut industry an estimated billion dollars, generated lawsuits for around thirty-five million dollars, and continued for over a year. We may also remember some other large ones, such as the 2006 recall of spinach and the 2008 one of peppers, and one or two of the ground beef or hamburger-associated recalls. But we never hear about the hundreds of others. Nor, I have noticed, do some retailers. Or at least they are not pulling those dangerous items off their shelves.

Another weakness in recalls is that they usually come too late—when the suspect food has already been eaten. Enough people have to become ill for anyone to pay attention. Even then, catching the culprit food and contaminant means backtracking it through the complex industrialized food system. This is a time-consuming investigation for the financially strapped government agencies that are responsible. It is also not unusual for an innocent food to be blamed first, while consumers happily keep eating the hazardous one. Remember when tomatoes were blamed for months for the outbreak caused by jalapeño and serrano peppers? Before that, there was the case of California strawberries blamed for an outbreak caused by Central American raspberries. More recently, poultry was initially suspected when peanut products were the culprit. It happens all the time.

Overall, food recalls are a mixed bag. It is all a matter of timing, good information—and cooperation by everyone right down the line to us.

In some instances—as noted in the chapters of this book—the industry has even taken the lead in promoting *additional* food safety measures. In other cases, the food industry and its associations—and the pharmaceutical or chemical industry—have fought against new regulations or changes, such as difficult-to-achieve higher standards, or restrictions on the use of a pesticide or hormone that is key to the industry's profits. New requirements that add to paperwork and delays, with no clear financial benefits, tend to be unpopular with the food industry.

One of the most important government-promoted measures in recent years, both in Canada and the United States, has been the forbiddingly named **Hazard Analysis and Critical Control Point** (HACCP) procedures. It has been progressively implemented in both countries since the 1990s. HACCP's goal is to help the food industry improve its safety measures and practices. The HACCP procedures I have looked at are really just a risk-based common-sense approach that helps food industry operations predict where safety problems are most likely to occur and make sure they don't happen. Well, at least *try* to make sure. The approach was used on NASA spaceflights back in the 1960s. Government took a long time to wake up to its potential. As long as it is applied properly, HACCP seems to be useful in our food supply as well. Of course, nothing will ever work completely. Food risks will continue.

3

There Are Smart Ways to Cut Your Food Risks

L ET'S RECAP. THERE are many kinds and sources of food hazards, and there is little evidence that our food risks are decreasing. Government regulators and any industry safety measures are not enough. Some of us are particularly likely to be seriously affected if we eat "bad food." *All* of us are at *some* risk of longer-term buildup of toxic substances in our body, which could contribute to those chronic health conditions that we all dread. True—often they won't show up for a while, but who wants to spend their "golden years" in a doctor's waiting room, staring at *People* magazine for hours? We'd rather be traveling, lunching with friends, playing golf or tennis, or pruning roses.

When it comes to what we eat, there is no such thing as "absolutely safe." But you *can* be safer. *The Safe Food Handbook* suggests smart decisions and actions that you can make every time you shop, cook, or eat, which can protect your health. No one will force you to do what is suggested. It is up to you to choose how safe you want to be. This book will help you choose what you want to do.

CHOOSE YOUR SAFETY LEVEL

◇ **Safety Level 1: You prefer to relax and ignore the whole food-safety issue.** Studies suggest that this decision is frequently made by teenagers and healthy adult males—until forced to change their mind. That is, if they think about it at all.

◇ **Safety Level 2: You believe you are moderately safe.** You are reasonably careful about what and how you eat, but do not go out of your way to choose low-risk foods.

◇ **Safety Level 3: You want to be safer.** This level suits health-conscious but currently healthy adults. You think of the safety aspect when you shop, prepare food, cook, eat out, or eat at home—but it is not the only deciding factor in what you do.

◇ **Safety Level 4: You want to be safest.** This is the super-safe choice—best if you have a high food-risk rating, or if you are an athlete or performer or otherwise need to be at your physical and mental peak at certain times. The safety of your food gets top priority.

But let me say a few things before I go any further. First, this book does not try to convince you to become a vegetarian or vegan, eat only organic, buy local, or join a community-supported agriculture (CSA) venture. All these suggestions are good, but they may not suit everyone. Even though they are not dogmatically advocated, you may find an implicit argument for them in the pages of this book. If your present eating preferences already fall into one of the preceding categories, you will find information that is relevant to you.

Second, as you will see in the text that follows, there is a great deal we still don't know about safety risks in our food, what causes them, what they will do to us, and how we can avoid them. Much of the longer-term research that is needed is difficult to do. To make matters worse, in a great many cases currently existing research is contradictory. In those instances, I have tried to summarize the arguments for both sides. This has not always been easy, as these are huge and specialized topics, and some of the original research that I reviewed was highly technical and rather mind extending. The secondary sources have often distorted the data to fit their particular bias. But at least you will be saved from plowing through all this mind-numbing information yourself. As an intelligent reader who knows your own risk rating, diet preferences, and time and budget constraints, you can make your own smart decisions about what is best for you to do. *You* can choose which research findings and which arguments to believe.

Third, I only *occasionally* urge that you stop eating some food item or other, simply because it is too high-risk. If such recommendations *are* made, they are usually specific to people in one or more high-risk groups, such as young children or pregnant women or those who have serious health conditions. Remember, too, that this book is about safety of food—not foods' nutritional side. Therefore, I do not make dietary recommendations based on nutritional arguments, such as avoiding trans fats or sugar.

Instead of advocating great dietary changes, this book suggests realistic—and often small—ways via which you can make safer food choices every time you shop, cook, and eat. It may change which tomato or lettuce you select or which fish you buy in a store or farmers' market. It could affect how you cook your potatoes or prepare your chicken dinner. It could alter the way you store your peanut butter, nuts, or fruit and when you throw out your unused eggs and yogurt. It may have some impact on what sushi or egg dish you order and what you ask to have put on your turkey sandwich. These are often mini-decisions. But they can have macro-consequences for your health.

As you read, you may also notice what could be called a certain recurring theme: Beware of *remote, raw,* and *ready.* That is because many of the risks that crop up in our breakfast, lunch, dinner, and snacks could be described by one or more of these terms (see sidebar).

FOODS TO THINK TWICE ABOUT— ESPECIALLY IF YOU HAVE A HIGH FOOD-RISK RATING

Remote—food that originates far from home, especially if from countries with polluted environments, questionable agricultural practices, and difficulty enforcing safety regulations.

Raw—and undercooked food, such as alfalfa, raw fish or shellfish dishes, undercooked meat and eggs, raw juices, and raw milk and raw milk cheeses. Unfortunately, those popular leafy greens and some wonderful fresh herbs can also be risky.

Ready—ready-to-eat foods that do not call for washing or cooking. They have usually gone through a number of stages, mixed products together, and been touched by a number of (maybe unwashed or contaminated) hands or equipment.

Will this book give you all the answers you ever want about risks in your food? No, it won't. Food safety is an enormous topic that could fill volumes. This book deals primarily with simple foods—fruits and vegetables, seafood, meat and poultry, dairy, eggs, grains, legumes, and nuts—and with contaminants that mainly get in unintentionally. Issues such as genetically modified (GM) foods and packaging materials are mentioned, but not discussed separately. These are huge, related topics on which other books are available (see page 317). Multi-ingredient, processed foods are also mentioned on occasions as relevant to the food group being discussed; however, a full discussion of the risks of processed foods is outside this book's focus. Many good books are available on topics such as preservatives, flavorings, coloring, and other key issues in food processing. The line had to be drawn somewhere.

Why are some contamination risks included and not others? The book focuses on health hazards in the North American food supply and the foods we like to eat in this part of the world. Having said this, I need to add that there are a few exceptions. Given the globalization of our food supply, population movements, and other factors, it is not impossible that parasites, certain currently rarely found bacteria and viruses, and very frightening threats such as **mad cow disease** (still cropping up in Canada at this time) will become more important issues here in the future. We need to be prepared. Just in case.

Why does the book deal with herbs and spices? When I began to look more into this issue, I realized how little we know about it—and how interesting the topic is. I have to confess that my own use—maybe even overuse—of herbs and spices also played a role. You may find that the topic is more relevant than you suspected. In fact, you may never look at that pepper shaker in quite the same way again.

A final word: Don't let concern about the safety of your food become a straitjacket, unless it really has to be. Food should be an enjoyable dimension of our lives—growing it, cooking it, and most of all, eating it. To quote Lubna Azmi: "A smart person knows all the rules so he can break them wisely." Unless you fall into one of the high-risk groups, just be sensible. Start where you can—and where you want to. Look at your risk rating and what you eat, and put the two together. Decide what you should do differently from what you are doing now, and take one step at a time. If you or a family member *does* have a high food-risk rating, then you will need to watch more carefully what you buy, and how you cook and eat. But always—enjoy.

4

Fruits and Vegetables

Unhealthy Produce?

IT SOUNDS LIKE slander. Just looking at that perfect red, delicately scented strawberry or that fresh piece of bright green broccoli makes me feel better. How can something that makes us healthy also hurt us?

But it can. And it is getting worse. Our fruits and vegetables are causing more and more big outbreaks of illness. In fact, according to statistics, *the largest number of food-related illnesses in the United States originates in fruits and vegetables.* There are now more produce-linked food-hazard-related outbreaks than are caused by poultry, beef, pork, or eggs. Seafood still tops the outbreak stakes, but almost four times as many people become ill from bad produce. We could even say that *fruits and vegetables are actually the most dangerous kind of food we eat.*

Remember the large *Salmonella* outbreak in 2006 that was associated with raw spinach, and the one in 2008, which started with fresh tomatoes as the suspect but was later found to have been caused by bacteria in imported jalapeño and serrano peppers? Just these two cases of contaminated produce together resulted in at least seventeen hundred confirmed illnesses. If we assume that only about 3 percent of actual cases may be reported and confirmed—which is quite likely—the number of resulting illnesses could be closer to fifty-seven thousand. And don't assume that these are just rare incidents. In between, and since then, we have had many less publicized outbreaks of food-borne illness linked to cantaloupe, corn, onions, strawberries, lettuce, and many other fruits and vegetables. Take one of our favorites, the tomato: since 1990 it has been guilty of at least fourteen major outbreaks in the American food supply. Often fresh diced tomatoes have been the culprit raw ingredient in one of our riskiest restaurant foods—salsa or guacamole.

Outbreaks are just the tip of the iceberg. Smaller incidents don't get publicized as an "outbreak," and most of the times we are ill, we remain blissfully unaware that "it was the lettuce that did it."

When we get a case of food poisoning from our produce, the usual cause is one or other invisible microorganism—often a bacterium, and less frequently, a parasite larva, a virus, or a mold (fungus). Vegetables are more likely to be contaminated than are fruit. Certain kinds of vegetables or fruit are riskier than others. In the final analysis, many factors are involved, including how we eat produce.

Nor is this the end of the story. Produce can also be the vehicle for longer-term health problems caused by toxic chemicals it carries, chemicals that form when we cook it, or even natural toxins. It is a fallacy that simply peeling the item protects us. *Any* kind of fruit or vegetable can prove to be the one we wish we hadn't eaten.

Why has produce become so dangerous? How is it getting contaminated? Who is to blame?

What Is Making Produce a High-Risk Food?

LET'S START WITH putting the blame on the industry. (I always prefer to blame someone else.) Most large-scale contamination of fresh vegetables or fruit starts on the farm. Our modern commercial food system has centralized production, with huge growers, processors, and distributors that generate and deliver tens of thousands of pounds of fruits and vegetables on any particular day. This system gives us the clean and perfect-looking produce we now expect: all items the same size and flawless—and yes, often pretty tasteless. Using masses of chemical fertilizers and pesticides helps.

A flawless appearance does not necessarily guarantee there are no microbes or toxic chemicals or other substances present. Organisms and chemicals attach themselves to fruit or vegetables not only while they are growing but also during the harvesting process, as well as postharvest, as fruit or vegetables are sorted, packed, transported, stored and often partially processed—often by peeling and cutting—for the RTE market. More handling equals more risk. And because huge distributors combine lettuce leaves or tomatoes or berries or whatever from several growers, one bad lot can end up contaminating others. Washing and refrigeration by producers, packers, or shippers may help for a while, but don't delude yourself—these processes rarely eliminate every microbe or trace of chemical. Don't forget, too, that it may be weeks before that tomato or strawberry reaches you. However they may have begun, problems spread. The small number of organisms that were there originally, which may not have been enough to hurt us, have had plenty of time to multiply from hundreds to thousands to tens of thousands and are now sufficiently numerous to make us ill. A pleasant living environment, and plenty of time—that is what microbes like.

That is just one side of the picture. I hate to admit it, but you and I are also helping to make our fruits and vegetables more dangerous to eat.

We are eating more of our produce raw. Think back to the last three times you ate fruit or vegetables. The chances are that you ate at least some of it raw—probably salad greens, coleslaw, tomatoes, carrots, celery, or green onions, and of course, fruit. You are not alone. Over the past few years we have started to eat more and more of our fruits and vegetables uncooked. In fact, close to 100 percent of American homes now serve salads. We also frequently consume salads when eating out. Fresh fruits and vegetables are good for us from a nutritional point of view. But from a safety perspective, eating raw produce carries many more risks. Raw produce has no cooking "kill" step that could deal with most of the contaminants that fruits and vegetables can carry, particularly those that have made their way right inside. Frozen vegetables are almost never involved in outbreaks, and frozen fruit only rarely. These days, canned produce is usually safe, too. The majority of produce-linked illnesses are caused by eating *fresh* fruit or vegetables.

We are buying more ready-to-eat fresh produce. Now, picture yourself in a supermarket produce aisle or even at your local deli, organic store, or co-op. See all those neat plastic bags and packages of prewashed and precut fruit or vegetables—salad greens, coleslaw, grated carrots, sliced apple, sliced pineapple, melon, and more. What you are looking at is evidence of the fast-growing multibillion-dollar RTE industry. **Fresh-cut produce** is the fastest-growing market segment within the fresh produce area. It is also the riskiest.

Stores are selling more and more of those neat little packages of produce because *we* want the convenience. Who wants to mess around peeling a cantaloupe or seeding bell peppers? But once fruit or vegetables are cut up, peeled, cored, and trimmed—or, from the produce point of view, "wounded"—microbes enter more easily. Think of it as being similar to a cut on your hand that can easily become infected. The invaders can come from the processing environment, from food workers (especially those who do the peeling and cutting if it is not done by machinery), from the equipment used, and even from packaging. Proportionally more outbreaks of produce-linked illness come from fresh-cut produce than from **fresh produce** that has been left whole. Some studies have concluded that cutting and slicing a fruit or vegetable *can multiply the contamination risk by six or more times.*

THAT LOVELY, FRESH, AND EASY BAGGED LETTUCE

Lettuce is one of the most popular bagged fresh produce products in America. Most Americans eat around thirty pounds of lettuce a year—most of it the least nutritious yet ubiquitous iceberg variety, although romaine is gaining in popularity. When you think how light lettuce is, that is a big mountain of greens. Nearly all the lettuce that is eaten in the United States is grown in two states—California and Arizona—almost year-round.

The modern food industry has brought this ancient vegetable up to the twenty-first century by turning it into a convenient RTE food. In fact, the largest growth in recent decades has been in the bagged, precut salad market, which is dominated by a few big firms. Now you have your choice: a whole head of unpackaged lettuce, washed heads of lettuce in sealed plastic bags, or "fresh-processed" washed and ready-to-eat shredded salad in a bag, sometimes with other greens and even the salad dressing and croutons thrown in.

The bagged lettuces look so nice and clean and safe. The precut kind saves time, and is triple prewashed (sometimes with added chemicals to make the washing more effective), right? So what is the problem? The problem is that bacteria can get right inside lettuce tissues, particularly when the leaves are cut. If the washing process is done well, it has been found to remove 90 to 95 percent of microbes. But, as government inspection records and outbreaks records show, enough *Salmonella* and *E. coli* bacteria can remain inside that crisp and clean bag to make us ill.

It was amazing that the outbreak in bagged, shredded romaine lettuce that resulted in product recalls in early May 2010 was ever identified and tracked down. It was caused by what the CDC calls "an emerging bacterial pathogen"—the very deadly **Shiga**-like toxin–

producing *E. coli* O145. This was the first time it had caused an outbreak in the United States—that we know of. Since only about 5 percent of U.S. laboratories apparently check for this *E. coli* serogroup (testing only for the familiar O157:H7), who really knows? The New York State Public Health Laboratory, which isolated and identified this bacterium in the bagged lettuce, has my admiration. Illnesses occurred in five states, with a very high hospitalization rate (around 40 percent), and with at least three victims who developed life-threatening kidney failure.

Just in the following two months, there was another huge recall of bagged salad greens because of *Salmonella* contamination and another due to *E. coli*—this time, for the more common *E. coli* O157:H7. So much for our "healthy greens."

We are eating more fresh produce in restaurants. Eating raw fruits and vegetables in restaurants is riskier than eating them at home. And yes, that sad-looking piece of lettuce and tomato with your burger or steak does count as produce. Yes, even that small, tasteless portion can carry enough "bad bugs" to make you sick. There—you have an excuse for not eating it.

We like to think salad bars offer healthy foods, but that may not be the case. The food usually sits there for hours, uncovered, waiting to be selected (my spot checks suggest that nine hours is not unusual), often with additional servings simply piled on top or stirred in when the aging remains run low. Flying insects, unclean utensils and serving vessels, other customers' hands and breath, scraps of contaminated items from nearby compartments, and poor temperature controls are common risk factors.

We are eating more imported produce. Do you remember when you used to eat only those fruits and vegetables that were in season? If not, your mother probably does. Now we want what we want whenever we want it, although that doesn't mean that we eat a wide variety. Even though we grow a lot of our own, nowadays, tens of billions of pounds of our fruits and vegetables come from countries such as Mexico, Chile, China, Honduras, Costa Rica, Guatemala, Brazil, and Ecuador. In the United States, close to half of fruit juices, almost half of fresh fruit, close to a fifth of fresh vegetables, and around a sixth of processed products such as dried fruits and frozen fruit are imported from other countries. This is about double what it was in the early 1990s. If you go buy fruit or vegetables in the following categories, there is a better-than-one chance in four that you will end up with produce that has been grown overseas.

- **Fruit:** avocados, bananas, blueberries, cantaloupe, grapes, honeydew melon, limes, kiwifruit, mangoes, papaya, pineapple, tangerines
- **Vegetables:** artichokes, asparagus, bell peppers, cucumbers, eggplants, garlic, radishes, squash, tomatoes

Is imported produce riskier? Research doesn't always agree. It seems to depend a great deal on the particular produce item, the time of the year (summers are worst), and which country it comes from (as in the case of all imports). Imported produce from some countries *does* appear to carry more contaminants, particularly those of human origin. In fact, the FDA found that imported produce was more than *three times* as likely to carry the dangerous *Salmonella* or *Shigella* bacteria than was domestic produce. In addition, the New York Academy of Sciences found norovirus and the hepatitis A virus to be much more common in imported fruits and vegetables. The academy also warns of completely new disease threats migrating to North America via imported fruits and vegetables. One example: Chagas disease, caused by a microscopic parasite, *could* enter through those wonderful açaí fruit juices from Brazil. (Don't you sometimes get the feeling that as soon as we find something gloriously healthy, it becomes unhealthy?)

There is also the issue of pesticide residues. We all know that several very toxic pesticides now banned in the United States and Canada are still in use in some of the countries from which we import produce. Correct usage is also difficult to control. I have often seen uneducated farmers in these countries simply operating on the "more is better" principle, particularly if working as farm laborers who aren't the ones paying for the pesticide used and haven't been instructed on proper use. The FDA seems to have acknowledged that imported fruits and vegetables are not only more likely to contain organisms that can cause serious illness but also more likely to carry illegal levels of pesticide. But this does not hold true in all cases, because a lot of factors are involved. Nor does it mean that our domestic produce is free from residues of toxic substances, either.

What We Eat

BY NOW WE don't need to be told that fruits and vegetables are an essential part of a healthy diet. They are a great source of vitamins, minerals, fiber, and antioxidants. Almost every day we hear something about a fruit or vegetable's role in preventing **cardiovascular** disease, high blood pressure, digestive problems, or cancer, or even helping us to lose weight. True, the reputation of the daily apple, as well as of spinach and broccoli, has faded, and the pomegranate and blueberry are no longer so much in the news. New and more exotic imported produce such as açaí and goji berries have taken their place, with even better promises. Which fruit or vegetable will it be tomorrow?

Although we know we should eat more healthy fruits and vegetables, we often don't do it. Not only are we eating too little, but most of us are also not eating the *best* fruits and vegetables. We can't blame availability. Thanks partly to hugely increased imports, there is an enormous range of fruits and vegetables to choose from in North America. But in practice most of us stick to a few favorites —year-round. Eating only the fruits and vegetables that are in season is hard to keep to—even for me, although I live in the great produce-growing state of California and like to think of myself as a **locavore**. I always want to have those avocados, tomatoes, blueberries, and bananas in my life, no matter the time of year.

Let's see how your favorite vegetables compare to those preferred by most people in North America: carrots, cabbage, lettuce, and white potatoes. Some that have been shown to be increasing in popularity are arugula, asparagus, bell peppers, corn, cucumbers, garlic, romaine lettuce, onions, squash, snap beans—and yes, even broccoli and spinach. We eat less of the healthiest dark green vegetables such as chard, mustard greens, and kale (try growing these yourself or buying locally grown—they will taste a lot better).

Although there are probably sixty or so different kinds of *fruit* to choose from in North American grocery stores, many of us stick to about six of them. Statistics show that the fresh fruits we eat the most are apples, bananas, grapes, oranges, and tomatoes. Increasing in popularity are avocados, blueberries, cherries, strawberries, tangerines, and such tropical fruits as mangoes, papayas, and pineapple.

DON'T BLAME THE TOMATO

It is believed that the tomato originated thousands of years ago in South America, probably Peru or maybe Bolivia. It was probably first domesticated by the Aztecs in Mexico. With the discovery of the New World, it was brought to Europe—Italy and Spain—and spread rapidly to other countries. Several different people, among them Thomas Jefferson, have been given credit for introducing tomatoes to North America during colonial times.

In some parts of Italy and North America, tomatoes were originally only used for ornamental purposes. People were afraid to eat them because they believed them to be poisonous, either because tomatoes belong to the nightshade family (as do peppers and white potatoes) or, more likely, because their acidic properties acted upon diners' pewter serving/dining ware, tainting the food with leached-out lead.

In our own day, it pays to be mindful of recipe instructions to prepare and store tomato dishes in "nonreactive" cookware and containers—such as glass, unscratched enamel, or stainless steel. We have passed the age of eating off pewter, but the fruit's acids can still cause a bitter-tasting (if not necessarily poisonous) reaction with aluminum ware.

As for the safety of those delicious fresh tomatoes? Well, at time of writing, the U.S. government has announced special "commodity-specific" guidance to the industry to help prevent microbes contaminating three of our riskiest foods. Guess what is on that list, along with leafy greens and melons? Well . . . tomatoes.

Who Keeps It Safe?

PRODUCE CAN BECOME contaminated in so many ways. Because we often eat it without cooking it, the need for safety oversight of raw fruits and vegetables is all the more important—more so than in the case of such foods as meat or poultry, which we eat cooked. Unfortunately, such regulations and inspections have been relatively neglected despite our increasing reliance on raw produce, RTE fruit and vegetable products, and imported produce.

The FDA is the main U.S. government agency responsible for keeping both our domestic and imported produce safe. The EPA also plays an important role in establishing tolerance levels for pesticide residues on our fruits and vegetables, based on their potential risk to human health, which the FDA then monitors. In Canada, fresh and processed produce is the responsibility of the CFIA. Among other things, it operates the priority-targeted National Chemical Residue Monitoring Program, which tests for a variety of contaminants in food, including agricultural chemicals, industrial and environmental pollutants, veterinary drugs (not relevant to produce), and even natural toxins.

Everyone—including the FDA—seems to agree that we need more comprehensive and effective oversight of fresh produce, including RTE fresh produce (that stuff in bags and on plastic trays). Because of budget constraints, plans for improvements have sat on the back burner for years. The FDA's involvement with the produce industry has been partial, and safety updates are often postponed. Inspection of firms that handle fresh produce only takes place every few years, which is far too infrequent. And, no meaningful on-farm inspection takes place.

In all, the FDA only spends about 3 percent of its food safety dollars and about 4 percent of its food safety staff time per year on fresh produce safety. Relate that tiny percentage to the important role that fruits and vegetables play in our diet. Yes, it is shockingly irrational. Things have improved a bit in recent years, but not enough and not fast enough. More resources have gone to preventing terrorist sabotage of our food supply (which is pretty well an impossible task) and to crisis-managing that constant stream of nasty outbreaks instead of to prevention.

I agree with those food safety experts who believe that the biggest safety gap in our produce is in *imported* produce. While the amount of imported produce, and its overall share in our diet, has been increasing rapidly over the past two decades, inspection has not kept up. Although imported fruits and vegetables may be inspected as much as nine times more frequently than domestic produce is, that is still not enough. In total, *less than 1 percent* of the billions of pounds of imported produce we eat each year will actually be checked at the border as it comes in—roughly one in every 134 shipments. Think of all the uninspected fruits and vegetables you are eating. . . .

Outsmarting Bacteria

Microbes are everywhere. Bacteria, mold, parasites, and viruses have taken up residence in your fresh fruits and vegetables more often than you think. Some are harmless, and others can make you very ill, particularly if you have a high food-risk rating. Testing of raw produce in the marketplace has found it to quite often carry *Salmonella*, *E. coli*, and *Listeria* bacteria. Actual findings of such studies vary, but as a very rough guide, you should assume that pathogenic bacteria could be present on, or in, your raw produce in one case out of ten. That is a frightening prospect.

Bacteria on fresh produce have caused many outbreaks of illness over the years. *Salmonella* or *Shigella* bacteria have turned up in raw apples, melon, cantaloupe, mangoes, lettuce, watermelon, strawberries, tomatoes, and orange juice. The dangerous *E. coli* O157:H7 has been linked to such fresh items as leaf lettuce, spinach, and strawberries, as well as to apple juice. Shredded cabbage has been found to hide bacteria that cause **botulism**. *Listeria monocytogenes* has been found in bagged ears of corn and in film-wrapped packages of perfectly nice-looking fresh mushrooms. These are only some examples.

As you now know, *E. coli* O157:H7 can be particularly dangerous for young children, as well as other vulnerable people. *Listeria monocytogenes* is a major risk to pregnant women and people with HIV/AIDS or other immune system–suppressing conditions (see page 185). *Salmonella* tends to be dismissed as just causing a few bad days with stomach cramps, diarrhea, and vomiting, but statistics show that at times it can be fatal, particularly to people over age fifty.

There are so many chances for bacteria to get in. Often—but not always—it takes places while produce is growing. In the field, common entry routes are water, soil, insects, soiled equipment, and wild or domestic animals roaming around the fields. Sometimes the source is people—especially in some of the poorer countries from which large quantities of our imported produce now come. When working on irrigation projects in such countries, I noticed that irrigation ditches frequently serve multiple functions, such as laundering and bathing, or worse—not just crop irrigation. No wonder the water is contaminated. Produce can also be contaminated by crop protection sprays or runoff that has passed through fields where those placid grass-fed, microbe-excreting cattle are grazing. A few incidents of imported contaminated produce, such as green onions, have been traced back to farmworkers' children defecating right in the fields (not a pleasant thought). Believe me, it happens. The culprits may also be insects or wild animals. Wild pigs were suspected in the 2006 case of spinach contamination (see sidebar), iguana lizards in a 2002 case of a *Salmonella* contamination of Mexican cantaloupes. Deer were the likely cause of a case of contaminated apple cider. Migrant birds and tree frogs may have been the perpetrators of several incidents of contaminated fruit on the East Coast. Even fruit flies can carry *Salmonella* bacteria. In our home garden, it could also be our own cat or dog.

Often the news media and even scientific publications give us an image of food contamination as a one-off incident. It may not be. In produce, it is more accurate to think in terms of levels of contamination going up and down and often up again (and sometimes down and up again). For instance, bacteria that enter while produce is growing may be mostly washed off afterward. But the few that are left behind can multiply, sometimes together with new ones that enter during processing. Their numbers may be reduced again during preparation and cooking in our home—or increased further during bad storage. After produce leaves the field, common risk factors include unsanitary equipment; careless harvesting procedures; contaminated transport containers or packing ice; people working in processing plants who may contaminate produce when washing, sorting, waxing, boxing, peeling, slicing, pulping, squeezing, drying, or shredding; . . . and our home.

Insects are common in the foods we eat, some entering in the field and others during storage or transport, or in the store. Like bacteria, many can multiply at an incredible rate. They can help to spread microbes while fruits and vegetables are in the warehouse or in the store, or even in our own kitchen (that ant, fly, or cockroach). Even the **processing water** used for washing the produce—supposedly to make it cleaner—can actually end up contaminating it, as in the famous mysterious mango incident of 1999 (see sidebar).

WASHING IN THE BUGS

We tend to think of washing our fruit or vegetables as a way of cleaning them and removing any contaminants. But the opposite can be true. It can actually "wash in" unhealthy microorganisms.

Washing is a normal part of fruit and vegetable production, processing, and marketing. During harvesting, washing is used to remove much of the soil and dirt that coats produce. Later on, it can be used to comply with export regulations, or to keep the produce fresh and attractive to buyers while it sits in the store. All this is fine as long as the *water* is clean.

One of the most puzzling produce-linked *Salmonella enterica* outbreaks in the United States, back in 1999, involved contamination of imported mangoes from Brazil. People in thirteen states became sick, some so ill that they had to be hospitalized. A few actually died. But the strange part was that mangoes from the same Brazilian grower were also shipped to Europe, where they made no one ill. Tests also showed that they were not contaminated, whereas the ones exported to the United States definitely were. How was this possible?

CDC investigators visited the farm that grew the mangoes. They found that those mangoes that were bound for America were dipped into unchlorinated hot water (about 115°F) for seventy to ninety minutes. After that, they were dipped into cold water. The purpose was to wash off any fruit fly larvae. This procedure was in line with U.S. import regulations. But unfortunately the water used was heavily contaminated with both *E. coli* and *Salmonella* bacteria. Because fruit is treated according to the regulations of the recipient country, the mangoes shipped to Europe were not given the water treatment. As a result, they did not become contaminated, whereas the ones sent to the United States did. Mystery solved.

But you are thinking, "Mangoes are peeled when they are eaten," right? Wouldn't this protect us? Apparently not. The researchers discovered that when warm fruit (not just mangoes, but even citrus fruits and tomatoes) are dipped into cold water, gases in the fruit contract and pull the bacteria from the skin right into the pulp. No amount of later washing, scrubbing, or peeling will get rid of them. Just to prove the point, a similar contamination occurred two years later, this time with mangoes imported from Peru.

The USDA has now recommended use of clean water and a waiting period between hot and cold treatments to avoid such problems.

We need to take better control of what happens in our own home. Once the fruit or vegetable is in our home, whatever bacteria load it carries will increase if we are not careful. New microbes can also enter fruit or vegetables through cross-contamination with other foods such as raw chicken or meat (see page 137). How quickly bacteria multiply also depends greatly on where, and at what temperatures, we store our produce. Of course, to obtain the greatest nutrient value from fruits and vegetables, we should eat them as soon as possible. But let's face it: Sometimes we simply can't do that. There are some generally agreed-upon principles about storing produce safely. But the source of our produce (supermarket, farmers' market, or home garden) and the condition we get it in (unripe and stored for weeks or fresh from the ground or tree) can also affect how long produce can keep. Sometimes we will also have to choose between taste and shelf life. This is one reason why there are so many differences of opinion on refrigerator versus room-temperature storage of produce.

Generally speaking, fruits and vegetables—like many other foods—need to be kept cool, dry, out of the sun, and away from insects. If unripe, many types of produce can just be kept at room temperature. But once they are ripe, refrigeration is best for many. (See sidebar on page 86 for specifics.)

Will "bad" bacteria in produce make us sick? Maybe, maybe not. It will partly depend on which ones are there, how many of them are present in what we eat, and our own personal risk level. In some cases the so-called **infective dose** of these powerful organisms is very small—perhaps one hundred to two hundred bacteria hiding in as few as five to ten "bad" berries or a few lettuce leaves. One or two mouthfuls could do it. With other bacteria, it will take more, particularly if we're a healthy adult. Those bacteria may not make us ill, but we will feel tired and run down as our body fights the invaders.

Some bacteria in or on produce do not even have to be present in the food to make us sick. The resistant toxins they leave behind are what could be dangerous. *Staphylococcus aureus,* which may get into foods from open wounds or the nose of food-service workers, can grow in certain foods and produce a toxin that causes intense vomiting. The disease we call botulism—which results in death in about 30 percent of cases—is caused by potentially lethal toxins of the bacterium *Clostridium botulinum,* which used to be common in poorly canned produce. Although it is relatively rare now, cases still occur, not just in home canning but even in large companies. An example is an established, family-owned canning company in Michigan that had to be repeatedly shut down by the FDA during 2008 because of possible *Clostridium* contamination in their cans of beans, peas, and asparagus.

Are there any safe fruits and vegetables? A number of factors could make one type of fruit or vegetable riskier than another, including how it grows, where it grows, and how we eat it. Nowadays, canned, frozen, and dried produce are safer from bacteria than is raw. FDA data tell us which have caused the most outbreaks of food-borne illness in the last twelve or so years, but this also has a lot to do with their popularity. Even if artichokes or endive were the most hazardous, they would not turn up in the statistics, simply because not enough people eat them to make the count. Also, let's remember that the list of most dangerous fruits and vegetables can change for a variety of reasons, including changes in our own eating patterns as well as in the contaminants involved.

Starting with the worst, these are the following current, common culprits: cabbage, carrots, grapes, green onions, lettuce, mangoes, melons, peppers, raspberries, snow peas, spinach, squash, and tomatoes. One of the largest and most publicized produce-linked outbreaks of the first decade of our twenty-first century was associated with spinach—not imported, but home-grown in California (see sidebar).

SPINACH CAN BE HAZARDOUS TO YOUR HEALTH

We tend to think of spinach as a superhealthy food. That is why the 2006 outbreak of the dangerous bacterium *E. coli* O157:H7 in bagged fresh spinach came as such a shock. During a period of a few months, at least 205 illnesses linked to spinach were confirmed in twenty-six U.S. states. More than one hundred people ended up in the hospital, and some thirty-one developed kidney failure (due to hemolytic uremic syndrome, or HUS). At least three people died. The dead included a two-year-old boy in Idaho.

When the outbreaks began to occur, the government food gum-shoes got busy. It soon became clear that fresh spinach was the prime suspect. The fact that illnesses were turning up in so many states suggested that the bacteria had entered early in the food chain—probably in the field where the spinach was grown. Investigators from the FDA, the CDC, and the affected states worked together to track down the farm or farms that the spinach came from.

Patients, growers, harvesters, and distributors were interviewed, data were collected and analyzed, and samples from victims were tested. A pattern emerged. Those who became ill reported having eaten prewashed raw spinach in bagged form. This narrowed things down a bit. On September 14, 2006, the FDA and the CDC held a conference call with the states and advised the public not to eat bagged fresh spinach until further notice. A number of companies that sold spinach under several different brand names put out broad voluntary recalls with a wide range of dates, just to make sure. To complicate things further, the FDA discovered that some retailers bought bagged spinach and then unbagged it. They had to expand the warning to include *any* raw spinach, as well as blended greens that contained fresh spinach.

Eat your spinach? Forget it. The poor vegetable was blacklisted. People began avoiding spinach, and many restaurants took spinach off the menu, whatever form it was in, raw or cooked.

Then the investigation got the sort of lucky break that every detective dreams of. Physical evidence turned up. On September 20, New Mexico's public health laboratory announced that it had isolated the outbreak's type of *E. coli* O157:H7 from an open package of spinach in the refrigerator of one of the victims (luckily the person had not cleaned out the fridge for a while). This was the "smoking gun," so to speak. Backtracking continued, to narrow the number of possible growers of the tainted vegetable. Eventually the list contained just four ranches in California, all of which used the same distributor.

But this was not the end of the mystery. How did the spinach become contaminated in the first place? It was important to answer this question so that another outbreak could be prevented. Now that the suspect farms were identified, the investigators got down to the basics. They spent many hours and days wandering around the fields and farms in the hot sun. They looked at how the spinach was watered, whether any animals came into contact with the fields where the leaves were grown, and watched how every step of harvesting and processing was done. One investigator was heard to say that he never wanted to eat spinach again as long as he lived.

But the actual cause was never identified. Although a number of suspects were considered, the prime one turned out to be a surprise— wild pigs. There were a lot of wild pigs on these farms, and they were actually observed at the scene of the crime, rooting around the growing crops. Tests showed their feces to contain the same dangerous bacteria as was found on the spinach. And where did the pigs get it from? Maybe from the cows in nearby yards. Or it could be that either the pigs, or the pigs and the cattle, somehow contaminated the groundwater, which then contaminated the spinach. Who knows? The outbreak is now in the food cold case files.

Organic produce is no safer from bacteria. At least, there is no convincing evidence that organic produce carries less bacteria than conventionally grown produce. You may know someone (like my former dentist, and one of my friends) who will happily eat an organic apple, lettuce leaf, or carrot without even washing it, claiming it is clean and safe. On the other side, we have those other people who argue that because organic growers use animal manure and other organic wastes that carry dangerous microbes, their produce will in fact be *more* likely to carry dangerous bacteria than conventionally grown produce. Some research I have looked at has certainly found this to be true. Naturally, the organic food industry disagrees. It points out that such risks are minimal because organic growers strictly adhere to the safety standards established by the USDA for manure composting and application. So which is right?

Many studies that have compared bacterial levels in organic produce with those in conventionally grown produce have found no significant difference. Look at these studies from a different angle. What they are telling us is that organic fruits and vegetables can be contaminated with bacteria (and parasites, and molds), just as can the foods' conventionally grown cousins. So while organic produce is presumably chemical free, don't just assume it is free of microbial contaminants.

Fruit juice can also be hazardous to your health. Let's take a quick look at this issue. Did you know that more than half of the fruit we eat is in the form of fruit juices? I suppose it is that convenience factor again: It takes a minute or two less time to gulp down a glass of orange juice than to peel or quarter four or five fresh oranges and eat them. Personally, I used to drink a lot of juice. Then I managed to revive a couple of half-dead orange trees in my backyard (and plant a few more) and discovered the pleasures of eating fresh oranges off the tree.

Overall, juices cause fewer cases of food poisoning than do fresh fruits and vegetables. But outbreaks do occur on a regular basis. A few years ago, the FDA estimated that each year there were between sixteen thousand and forty-eight thousand cases of juice-related illnesses in the United States. *E. coli, Salmonella,* and *Cryptosporidium* bacteria have been found in apple juice; *Salmonella* and *Bacillus cereus* bacteria have turned up in orange juice; and even carrot juice has carried dangerous *Clostridium botulinum* bacteria.

Most of these outbreaks trace back to raw juices—not those boring pasteurized supermarket juices, often based on imported juice concentrates from thousands of miles away (China now accounts for over half of the apple juice sold in the United States). Even if the fruit used is picked off the ground or otherwise contaminated, pasteurization of the juice will kill most bacteria. Although commercially sold unpasteurized raw juices and cider account for only about 2 percent of the U.S. market, most cases of juice-linked food poisonings occur in these. These are the type of juices you buy from a vendor at the farmers' market, who keeps it in an icebox, or from the refrigerated section of a grocery or health-food store. They tend to be riskier than the fresh-made ones you can get in juice bars or some restaurants or make in your own home. If freshly squeezed juices are left untreated, even for a short time, the harmful bacteria that were inside the fruit, or even on the outside, can rapidly increase in numbers. Yes, these juices taste a great deal better than pasteurized ones, and if uncontaminated are healthier for us, but they can also be dangerous. We used to think that the acid in juice would kill any organisms, but we now realize that isn't always true. They are far too hardy.

If unpasteurized raw juices are so dangerous, why are they still being sold? Whenever bans on raw juice have been proposed, there has been public outcry. This, together with industry pressure, have made it difficult to ban them completely. But regulations *have* been tightened. Any commercially sold unpasteurized juice in the United States is now supposed to carry a warning label such as the below:

> WARNING:
> This product has not been pasteurized and therefore may contain harmful bacteria that can cause serious illness in children, the elderly, and persons with weakened immune systems.

Canada is also taking steps to reduce illnesses from unpasteurized juices or cider. Known producers and their products are monitored and encouraged to use a code of practice to make their products safer. They are also advised to label their products "unpasteurized."

But you can still buy raw juices—as well as make them yourself, which is the safest form. Juices that are sold by the glass do not have to comply with this regulation. Juice bars are exempt. So are restaurants that make fresh juices. And—you will be pleased to know—so is your child's lemonade stand. And take a look next time you buy unpasteurized juice: you will see that the warning label is difficult to find, and often isn't there at all.

Some states, such as New York, have passed safety measures that make the legal sale of unpasteurized juice virtually impossible. But as in the case of buying raw milk (see page 188), if you really want it, you can always find a way. Maybe you can just claim you are buying it to make cider wine (and sign a form that says that), which can make it legal in many places. But now some formerly raw-juice companies have started to pasteurize their juice products, after almost being bankrupted by outbreaks. Odwalla, Inc. (formerly a private company based in California, but now a subsidiary of Coca-Cola) is a case in point. After a very costly *E. coli* O157:H7 contamination of its raw apple juice in 1996, which resulted in a 90 percent reduction in sales, the company switched to using flash pasteurization.

KNOW YOUR JUICES

◇ **Pasteurized juice:** Pasteurization kills most bacteria by exposing them to high heat for a short period of time. This is the type of juice you are most likely to buy in the supermarket.

◇ **Flash-pasteurized juice:** This process differs from the usual pasteurization in that the juice is treated with a higher heat for only 15 to 30 seconds. It is supposed to better maintain the color and flavor. Some of the popular commercially sold brands of juice, kept in a separate refrigerator, which you think are raw juice, are nowadays actually flash-pasteurized (often stated in very fine print on the label, where you unlikely to even notice it).

◇ **Treated juice:** The juice you will see in a farmers' market or health food store, sometimes marketed as "fresh squeezed," may be labeled "treated" instead of "pasteurized." If done properly, by such methods as approved by the FDA (for instance, UV irradiation), most bacteria would be destroyed. Unfortunately, this is not always the case.

◇ **Untreated or raw juice:** These juices have received no treatment to kill microbes. Although they have a committed following among those who believe in the superior nutritional value of raw juice and prefer the much better taste, they are not recommended for people in high-risk groups.

Evading Toxic Molds

CERTAIN MOLDS (FUNGI) on food can, when the conditions are right, produce carcinogenic toxins. That is the bad news. The good news in the case of fruits and vegetables is that if we are careful, we can largely avoid them.

We have all seen mold on fruit or vegetables at some point, and probably on other foods as well: fuzzy green dots on stale bread, frightening black fuzz in that container of sour cream that we were about to put on a baked potato, furry growth in that jar of jelly or creamed corn that got lost in the back of the refrigerator, white dust on outdated Cheddar . . . and round velvety green, gray, or white circles or fuzz on fruit. The problem is that molds and their spores are everywhere in our environment and can so easily get into our food. Although molds prefer to grow in warm and moist conditions, they can also grow at refrigerator temperatures. Moldy foods can have invisible bacteria growing alongside them.

Some molds, including many found on our fruits and vegetables, are harmless except to sensitive people for whom they can give allergic reactions or trigger respiratory conditions. The most dangerous molds for all of us are those that produce poisonous **mycotoxins** when the conditions are right. Several of these mycotoxins have been associated with increased risk of several forms of cancer, and with a range of other diseases as well. The research is in its infancy, so we are finding out more unpleasant things all the time. There are about three hundred of these toxins, and more are being discovered. Some of the most common ones are: aflatoxin, **fumonisin, Vomitoxin,** zearalenone, and ochratoxin. These mycotoxins are not limited to produce. They can be found in many of our foods, including tree nuts, peanuts, grains, spices, and even dairy. The molds that produce them when the conditions are right include strains of the fungi *Aspergillus, Claviceps, Fusarium,* and even *Penicillium*. In produce, such mycotoxin-producing molds can occur on a wide range of items. They can enter in the field, during storage, or in our own kitchen. The Food and Agriculture Organization of the United Nations (FAO) estimates that as much as 25 percent of the world's food crops may be affected by mycotoxins.

How do we know which moldy berry, apple, or papaya is safe to eat, and which we should avoid? We don't. Molds are difficult to tell apart if one is not an expert, and we can't tell by looking at a mold if it is producing toxins or not. Given these problems, the safest approach is to avoid eating *any* molds at all (unless they are those good ones in your favorite cheeses). But don't assume that just cutting off the moldy part of a raspberry or apple or zucchini will eliminate the risk. The problem is that mycotoxins can spread throughout the fruit or vegetable, far beyond the mold that we see, especially if the item is soft. Correct storage (see page 86) is very important for avoiding molds as well as other spoilage organisms.

As in the case of bacteria, how badly a mycotoxin such as aflatoxin will affect someone depends on how much of which toxin is present, how much of the mycotoxin-laden food has been eaten, and how susceptible the person is. Because of government controls in North America, we don't need to worry about acute aflatoxicosis from a large dose. But longer-term exposures to low levels of several of these mycotoxins from several of our foods, including from produce, may be much more relevant. There are plenty of alternative medicine solutions on the market for ridding our food or body of them. Unfortunately, there is no scientific proof that any of these remedies work. So skip purchasing them—and concentrate on avoiding molds in the first place (see sidebar).

That isn't easy. Personally, I am convinced that mycotoxins in our food are one of the biggest health risks presently facing us in the developed world. They could well be the cause of not just many cancers but of several other mysterious conditions of children as well as adults. My concern probably has something to do with my years of research on fungi. It also has to do with the fact that molds are everywhere, so insidious, so difficult to avoid. And, we know so little about the longer term effects of small yet regularly ingested amounts of such toxins.

HOW TO AVOID MOLDS

The best way to avoid mold growth in your home is to keep humidity low (below 40 percent). If there is a musty smell, it usually means that there is mold hiding somewhere. To prevent the contamination of food by mold spores:

◇ Keep covered any food that you are waiting to serve, to block entrance of mold spores from the air.
◇ Don't leave any perishable foods out of the refrigerator for longer than two hours.
◇ Throw out any moldy food you find in the refrigerator and wash the refrigerator with a bleach solution (try one part bleach to one part warm water—but watch your eyes!)

◇ Empty any leftover canned food into clean storage containers and refrigerate promptly.

◇ Use leftovers within three to four days.

◇ Wash used dishes, cutlery, and cooking utensils and pans promptly.

◇ Generally, keep your kitchen clean and dry (see page 89).

Unwelcome Parasites

PARASITES IN NORTH American food? Yes, unfortunately they are not nearly as rare as we like to think. There are hundreds of thousands of different kinds of parasites, and—like molds and bacteria—they are everywhere, including on our fruits and vegetables.

No, the issue here is not that rather cute-looking smiling green worm, often shown in illustrations in the act of popping out of a bright red apple. Parasites are much meaner—and uglier. By definition, they are small or even microscopic organisms that live off their host, without contributing anything in return. (It sounds rather like the definition of a teenager.) According to the World Health Organization (WHO), about a quarter of the world's population carries around chronic intestinal parasites. Infection in North America is believed to be lower, but it's still much higher than statistics show—and than we like to think.

Two common ways we can catch parasites is by not washing our fresh vegetables or certain fruit properly, and by eating out at places where food handlers don't use good hygiene (many of our food workers unknowingly carry the critters). But true, we can also catch them in other ways, such as during international travel, from our pet, or even from our significant other. Many of the parasites that sneak into our fruits and vegetables can be traced back to irrigation water contaminated with *human* (not animal) feces. Imported produce tends to be the most exposed to such contaminated water, particularly when it comes from hot climates where certain parasites are widespread among the farming population. Testing has shown high levels in places such as Central America and South America—where a lot of our berries originate. But at times, high levels of parasites have also been found in irrigation water in North America.

If you have ever had a parasite—and I have had several—you will know that they rarely kill you but can make you thoroughly miserable for as long as forty days. They can also leave you with longer-term health issues such as chronic digestive problems, fatigue, damage to your immune system, and even end up in your liver or in your brain (It is a toss-up which is worse). Some parasites in particular are very difficult to get rid of once they are in your body.

Dismissing parasites as no longer relevant in such countries as the United States and Canada is a mistake. There is plenty of evidence to argue that at least some of these parasites are on the increase, whether they are brought in or originate here. Our love of raw fruits and vegetables (and fresh herbs) is one of the reasons. Globalization of our food supply is another. Imported foods are more likely to carry them. So are food-service workers from other countries.

The parasites in our fresh fruits and vegetables are usually minute **protozoan** parasites (very small one-celled organisms) such as *Giardia, Cyclospora* (see sidebar), *Cryptosporidium,* and *Toxoplasma gondii.* They are likely to hide in such fruit as berries, as well as in fruit salad, raw (unpasteurized) juices and apple cider, and leafy vegetables. In recent outbreaks, *Giardia lamblia*—a particularly persistent parasite that I know well—has been linked to eating raw vegetables, raw fruit, and food from salad bars. *Cryptosporidium* has caused illnesses through its presence in apple cider and organic lettuce. Several other protozoa, including *Glaucoma* spp., *Tetrahymena* spp., and *Colpoda steinii,* have also turned up in our lettuce and spinach.

CYCLOSPORA COULD BE AN EMERGING FOOD RISK

Cyclospora cayetanensis is now one of the most common food-borne parasites in America—and an emerging problem. It is a tiny one-celled parasite, originating in Papua New Guinea. As little as a decade ago it was virtually unknown here, which shows how quickly the situation can change. This parasite has been linked to outbreaks in such produce as lettuce, raspberries, blackberries, strawberries, green beans, and fruit and vegetable salads, as well as to several other foods—even raw milk.

The number of U.S. cases has dramatically increased in the past decade. It is believed that many of us now host this parasite in our body—without knowing it. One of the devious features of *Cyclospora* infection is that it does not cause symptoms in everyone. You or I could become a carrier and pass it on to others. The rapid spread is believed to be helped by the number of carriers now working in our **food-service industry**.

Outbreaks of *Cyclospora* usually occur in late spring or early summer. This is also the time of year when we import a lot of fresh fruits and vegetables from our southern neighbors. Berries seem to be one of the riskiest foods. The biggest upsurge of *Cyclospora* infections in the United States occurred in the late 1990s, when we had several outbreaks and over two thousand identified cases. The larger outbreaks were linked to Guatemalan raspberries that had probably been irrigated with feces-contaminated water. These outbreaks virtually destroyed the Guatemalan berry industry. Initially California strawberries had been the suspect, resulting in some forty million dollars in losses to the strawberry industry. But not all outbreaks in produce have been caused by imported raw produce. Some of the smaller outbreaks have originated right here in the United States.

Some outbreaks suggest that a person can eat as few as half a dozen contaminated berries and still get sick.

If you live in North America and pick up a parasite from your food, there is a good chance that you will not be correctly diagnosed. The vague symptoms (loss of appetite, weight loss, nausea, gas, stomach cramps, muscle ache, vomiting, low-grade fever, bloating, and fatigue) are very similar to other diseases such as irritable bowel syndrome (IBS) and the flu. Doctors with only limited training in parasitology are likely to think of these first, and even if ordered, laboratory tests are unlikely to be properly done for a number of reasons.

Cruising with a Virus

ALTHOUGH THEY DON'T hit the news as much as bacteria, roughly half of produce-linked outbreaks in recent years have been caused by viruses. Whereas bacteria often contaminate produce while it is growing, viruses tend to enter at later stages. They are also more likely to have a human cause. Many smaller outbreaks take place in private homes, with only a few illnesses. Others affect tens or hundreds of people and occur in such places as restaurants, banquets, institutional settings, workplaces, and even bowling alleys— anywhere people gather and eat the same food, particularly if it is mass prepared, and sits around for a while. Viruses are most likely to contaminate fresh fruit or vegetables, although they have also been found in frozen fruit.

The majority of documented incidents of food-borne viral outbreaks have been traced to items that had been handled manually by an infected food handler and that were then eaten raw.

The same problem exists with viruses as with parasites— diagnosis is difficult and a large percentage of cases are never linked to food. Again, symptoms such as bad diarrhea, nausea, violent and sudden vomiting, and cramps are often mistaken for "stomach flu."

Norovirus (which used to be called "Norwalk-like virus"; see sidebar) is by far the most common viral food contaminant. Hepatitis A virus (which affects the liver, and is certainly not something you want) also occurs frequently as a contaminant of fruit or vegetables.

As in the case of bacteria, virus contaminants are more likely to be associated with certain fruits and vegetables than others, and are more common in imported produce. Hepatitis A has partnered with such foods as green onions and scallions (quite common), lettuce (also common), cabbage, celery sticks, potatoes, salads, and frozen or fresh raspberries and strawberries. Norovirus has turned up in such produce as bananas, beans, broccoli, cantaloupe, grapes, pineapples, raspberries, and strawberries. It has also appeared in coleslaw; fruit, potato, and vegetable salads; guacamole; onion rings; and more. Frozen rather than fresh berries have been involved in a few cases. Greens-based salads and lettuce are particularly popular with norovirus. Salad dressings often give a helping hand.

THE CRUISE SHIP VIRUS

The CDC believes norovirus causes as many as 50 percent of all cases of food-borne outbreaks in the United States. It is extremely infectious, resistant to freezing, and can even survive disinfection of countertops with alcohol-based disinfectants or detergents. It only takes low numbers of norovirus to make someone ill. Symptoms can develop within a day of exposure and last for several days. Usually the illness is relatively mild, but at times it can be so severe that it lands seemingly healthy people in intensive care.

Norovirus seems to have a particular affinity for places where we are supposed to be having a good time, such as wedding receptions, restaurants, and cruise ships. There are several recorded cases of its turning up in the fresh fruit filling of wedding cakes. (Maybe James Thurber was right after all when he said, "The most dangerous food is wedding cake.") But norovirus turns up frequently in less entertaining, densely populated institutional settings as well, such as nursing homes, jails, army bases, and even medical conferences. Large outbreaks of norovirus have been traced to food that was handled by just one person.

Norovirus is a cruise ship nightmare. (If you are about to go on a cruise, perhaps you should skip this paragraph.) There have been numerous outbreaks of this bug on cruise ships. Accounts of these outbreaks actually make quite interesting reading (if you enjoy forensics or if other people's misery comforts you). In many cases, hundreds of both passengers and crew members have become ill. In one odd case, almost half the crew was stricken while the passengers, who did not become ill, had to fend largely for themselves for the rest of the trip. Not what you would call a luxury cruise.

Cutting Down on Pesticide Residues

MANY OF US worry about ingesting pesticide residues from fruits and vegetables. There is a very good chance that we do—even if we eat organic produce, although it's less likely there. But just how harmful are the relatively small amounts we are getting? And what produce items can we safely eat?

Amazing though it may seem, after all these years of pesticide use, we still don't have a good answer. Research on health effects simply cannot keep up with the thousands of different pesticides in use. Let's face it, pesticides are harmful by design. If they kill bugs, rodents, weeds, and mold, why expect them to have no effect on us? True—the human body is a lot bigger than that of a fruit fly, but then, unlike the already short-lived pests such substances are meant to dispatch before their time, we are being exposed to them year after year, and many of them build up in our body over time.

More than twenty thousand pesticide products are registered in the United States alone. The EPA registers them and sets maximum tolerances for their presence. Levels are monitored by the FDA and USDA/FSIS. This is not a static situation. New pesticides are added all the time, established tolerances are periodically reviewed—and maybe revised. The worst pesticides are gradually phased out. In other words, they are "safe" until they are defined as unsafe.

COMMON KINDS OF PESTICIDES

Pesticides are chemical or biological products that have been developed with the purpose of controlling weeds, insects, fungi, diseases or other pests on crops, animals, or buildings and outdoor living areas such as parks and gardens. The most common pesticides are:

◇ **Fungicides:** used to control molds or fungi
◇ **Herbicides:** used to control weeds
◇ **Insecticides:** used to control insects
◇ **Molluscicides:** used to control slugs and snails
◇ **Rodenticides:** used to control rats and mice

All these types of pesticides may be used during food production as well as at later stages, to protect food from pests while it is stored and transported.

Even if we don't yet have the final answer about risks, given a choice, pesticide residue is not something you and I want. But can we escape it? During the last fifty years, pesticides have come to be very widely employed everywhere. As resistance grows among plant pests, larger and larger applications are used to protect growing fruits and vegetables against weeds, insects, and mold. Again, our industrialized food supply plays a role: Many pesticides are used to slow down spoilage and ripening postharvest, while fruits and vegetables from far away are en route to our table. True, such use increases productivity, reduces losses, and sometimes has other safety benefits (as when pesticide use kills insects that carry bacteria or mold). And, yes, this means cheaper food for us.

Safety measures are in effect. Maximum residue limits (MRLs) for many toxic substances in pesticides now restrict the amount of such residues that can "safely" remain in or on our food. And again, the most toxic agricultural pesticides are progressively being banned or tolerances adjusted once research shows that they have been too lax. At the same time, according to CDC and other testing, most of us are walking around with detectable levels of a toxic chemical cocktail in our body, not all but probably much of it from our food. No one seems to really know what the cumulative or synergistic effects may be over the longer term. Or how it is shortening our life span.

As mentioned earlier, food can't be blamed for all of the chemical residues in our body. We are exposed to a number of sources every day of our lives. Pesticides are also used in homes, places of business, schools, parks, hospitals, and so on. Even if our food is just one contributor of toxic chemicals, and even if the amounts are relatively small, it adds to our total body burden.

So how often are there pesticide residues on our fruits and vegetables? Estimates range from around 35 to 76 percent. Let's just say that low levels of pesticide residues may be found in *most* fresh fruit or vegetables, as well as in juice or other processed produce products.

How much pesticide residue we are getting from our fruits and vegetables will depend on several factors, including where the produce comes from, whether it is conventionally grown versus organic, and which fruit or vegetable we are eating. Just looking at a single vegetable such as, say, a carrot, there can be enormous differences in the pesticide levels of the carrots grown in the United States and those grown in Canada (some tests have found Canadian carrots to have twelve times' higher levels of DDT residues—but these are not recent data).

We are likely to be more at risk for pesticide residues from imported produce than we are from home-grown, although this does not always hold true. Most countries do have some type of government control of pesticides. But such regulations can be poorly enforced. Not surprisingly, it has been found that imported fruit are *four times* more likely to carry dangerous amounts than U.S.-produced ones, and imported vegetables twice as likely. Of course, it varies. And this may be an overestimation. But the general comparison is most likely true. On occasion, imported fruits and vegetables are also found to be contaminated with residues of extremely dangerous pesticides that are now banned in the United States.

Yes, organic fruits and vegetables have less chemical pesticide residue. Production and storage of certified organic fruits and vegetables use far fewer and less chemical fertilizers and synthetic pesticides than do conventional alternatives. To get rid of pests, **organic farming** substitutes naturally occurring and safer substances such as sulfur, oils, soaps, copper, certain microbial pesticides, *Bacillius thuringensis,* and pheromones. (There are not necessarily substances we want in our body, either, but at least they are natural!)

Research has proved what we always believed—that our body is less likely to get a load of unhealthy chemicals from organic fruits and vegetables than from nonorganic ones. But very small amounts of chemical pesticide residue *can* exist in organic produce as well. Why? Such residues could come from previous land use, contaminated irrigation water, pesticides in rain or groundwater, chemical sprays drifting from neighboring nonorganic farms, mixing or mislabeling of produce, last-resort efforts to get rid of pests in organic production, or plain deceit. But even so, it is estimated that organic has only about a fifth of the pesticide residues of conventional produce. Such amounts are too small to worry about.

So if you want to reduce your exposure to pesticide residues, eating organic produce is a good idea. But you may have to pay as much as 50 percent more for organic produce, unless you are buying it in season at a farmers' market or grow your own. To keep to your food budget, you may want to be selective and shop organic only for items likely to carry the heaviest pesticide load (both because they are sprayed the most, and because they retain the residues). That is, provided you don't have special sensitivities to chemicals. Thanks to research by the USDA laboratories, the Institute for Agriculture and Trade Policy (IATP), and the Environmental Working Group (EWG), we do have some idea of which ones these are (see sidebar). However, note that not everyone completely agrees with this classification of worst and safest, and it can also change over time.

In general, softer-skinned fruits and vegetables are likely to carry more residues than those with thicker and tougher skins. Wouldn't you know it, those delicious peaches seem to be the worst fruit, and nectarines and strawberries are close behind. Some studies have found almost all conventionally grown peaches to test positive for pesticide residues. Some tests of a single sample of strawberries or blueberries have found as many as thirteen different pesticide residues. Sweet bell peppers and that innocent-looking celery are leaders among the pesticide-contaminated vegetables. Usually multiple different chemicals have been found to be present. According to some reports, imported cucumbers are close behind, but for some reason, they were not placed on the "worst" list.

EATING ORGANIC ON A BUDGET

According to www.foodnews.org, these are the "dirty dozen" of the produce world—the ones to buy "organic," whenever possible:

◇ peaches, strawberries, apples, blueberries, nectarines, cherries, imported grapes, celery, bell peppers, spinach, kale/collard greens, and potatoes.

The fifteen cleanest types of produce (in terms of pesticide residues, but not necessarily other contaminants)—which you can buy "conventional" to protect your budget:

◇ Onions, avocado, sweet corn, pineapple, mangoes, sweet peas, asparagus, kiwi, cabbage, eggplant, cantaloupe, watermelon, grapefruit, sweet potato, and honeydew melon.

If you just look at fruits and vegetables in terms of residues of those particularly toxic pesticides such as DDE (a soil metabolite of DDT), or dieldrin, the ranking could be different. The Pesticide Action Network has listed the following produce items (in alphabetical order) as among the most dangerous pesticide-residue foods we eat. Let's call them the "superdirty six":

◇ cantaloupe, cucumber, radishes, spinach, summer squash, winter squash

You will notice if you compare the sidebar with the above list, that cantaloupe is on both the "super-dirty six" list and the "safest" list. The reason could lie in the fact that the "safest" list tested domestic cantaloupe, whereas the other research may have tested an imported sample. Source has a lot to do with safety. I have also read research that puts carrots on the "superdirty six" list. But again, there were wide differences according to where the carrots were grown. Nevertheless, that is one of the reasons I decided to plant some this year, although I am not sure it will do much good. Trouble could be there, lurking in my own backyard. Root vegetables may pick up such residues even if they are not sprayed, if the soil has been contaminated at some earlier point in time.

If you have to make a choice within your family as to who gets organic and who gets conventional produce, you may want to give priority to your children, and to yourself if you are pregnant, because of higher risks. Some CDC tests show that American infants and children already carry frighteningly large amounts of toxic chemicals in their body. Supporters of synthetic pesticide use in agriculture argue that our children will have more exposure to pesticides from a day in the schoolroom, a crawl around the playroom carpet, or a walk in the park. But research suggests that their food may be a significant or even a greater risk factor. Studies that have compared children who ate a mostly organic diet with those who ate a conventional diet found much lower body levels of pesticide residues in children who ate organic. Looking at the cumulative picture, it would make sense to at least control what you can.

Even small doses of pesticide residues that would not harm an adult can result in permanent damage to infants and young developing children because their nervous system, brain, and endocrine and reproductive systems are still developing. A few studies have found higher instances of diseases such as leukemia and brain cancer in children with high early exposure to pesticides. An additional risk factor for infants is the fact that they consume very few kinds of fruits and vegetables and related products, such as apple juice, applesauce (apples have been found to be one of the most pesticide-contaminated fruits—see sidebar, page 66) and orange juice. That is, even if the produce you give your child contains a very low level of a toxic chemical, if it is eaten repeatedly the child is going to get quite a bit over the course of a month or a year, particularly in terms of his or her body weight.

Remember those highly toxic pesticides such as DDT, chlordane, and others that were considered safe right up to the day that the EPA banned them? Several more will be phased out over the next few decades, because of health risks—but at a frustrating snail's pace. By the time some of these dangerous ones are finally banned (with industry fighting every step of the way), we will have already been exposed to them for years or even decades. The toxic pesticide lindane, which can cause cancer and disrupt the hormone system, is an example. In 2006, the EPA finally withdrew lindane from all agricultural use after close to half a century of use in the United States, with thousands of reports of illness and some reported deaths and after at least fifty-two other countries had banned it long ago.

What can we do in the meantime? Apart from making smart produce choices, we can wash and peel. Research has found that if we wash well with tap water, we can reduce the levels of about three out of four pesticides. And if we use commercially sold fruit or vegetable washes? Testing of washes on such produce as lettuce, tomatoes, and berries shows that they *don't* help. So save your money.

Avoiding Natural Toxins

MOST FRUITS AND vegetables contain small amounts of natural toxins. It is believed that some plants rather cleverly use such substances as a kind of a built-in natural pesticide to protect themselves against insect attacks. If you eat these fruit or vegetables in moderation, no problem. However, a few produce items contain toxins that could make you very ill, even in smaller quantities (see sidebar). The good news about the natural toxins—unlike many other dangers in our food—is that we can usually avoid them.

SOME FRUITS AND VEGETABLES WITH DANGEROUS NATURAL TOXINS

Potatoes: Potatoes contain low levels of natural toxins called glycoalkaloids, also known as saponins, which can cause headaches, stomach upset, vomiting, and even cause death. They are not destroyed by cooking. These levels are usually higher in green parts of the potato, in the eyes, in potato sprouts, and in the peel. Be particularly careful to remove any green or damaged sections before you cook, or toss the potato entirely if the skin is green-tinged. Avoid eating potatoes that taste bitter.

Cassava: Raw or unprocessed cassava (yuca) contains a naturally occurring toxin called cyanogenic glycosides. It can cause breathing difficulties, paralysis, staggering, and can be fatal. Peel, slice and cook cassava thoroughly (bake, boil, or roast). Treat frozen cassava the same way.

Rhubarb: The leaves of the rhubarb plant contain a harmful toxin called oxalic acid. Oxalic acid poisoning can cause muscle twitching, cramps, decreased breathing and heart action, vomiting, pain, headache, convulsions, and coma. Even potentially fatal kidney damage can result. Do not eat rhubarb leaves, only the stems. (Stores often sell rhubarb with at least part of the leaf attached. Remove it before cooking, right down to the point where there is no leaf at all.) Vegetables such as spinach, Swiss chard, beet, collards, okra, leeks, and several other fruits and vegetables (as well as some nuts, legumes, and grains), also contain lower levels of oxalic acid (usually higher in the leaves than in the root, stem, or stalks). The body can deal with small amounts, but large amounts of this substance (for instance, from eating several pounds of spinach) can be toxic. Oxalic acid is believed to inhibit absorption of calcium from the plant itself (calcium absorption from other foods that are eaten at the same time is apparently not affected).

Fruit pits and seeds: Peach, apple, pear, cherry, plum, and apricot seeds, shoots, and twigs contain the glycoside amygdalin. When hydrolized (a chemical process that takes place in the body), amygdalin produces hydrogen cyanide. Do not eat them.

Kumara: When kumara (a member of the sweet potato family) is injured or attacked by insects, it can produce toxins, the most common of which is ipomeamarone, which produces a bitter taste when eaten. Cut away any damaged sections, and do not eat sweet potatoes that taste bitter.

Parsnips: When parsnips are stressed or injured, they can produce a group of natural toxins known as furocoumarins, which can result in severe stomachache. The levels of these toxins are usually highest in the peel and near the damaged area. Peel parsnips before cooking and discard any cooking water.

Zucchini: Zucchini can sometimes contain natural toxins known as cucurbitacins, although rarely if commercially grown. Eating such zucchini has caused people to experience stomach cramps, vomiting, diarrhea, and collapse. Do not eat zucchini that taste bitter or have a strong, unpleasant smell.

Wild Mushrooms: Poisonous mushrooms grow almost anywhere. They are hard to tell from nonpoisonous ones. Children (and pets) are most vulnerable. Mushroom toxins are not inactivated by cooking. Effects can range from the sudden but short-term gastrointestinal upset caused by Green Gill, Sickener, Pepper Bolete, Horse Mushrooms, and Tiger Top, to the much more dangerous effects of the group of mushrooms that includes Fool's Mushroom, False

Morel, Destroying Angel, and Death Cap. Some of the most dangerous mushrooms are lethal about 50 percent of the time, and if you do survive, recovery will usually take months. Inky Cap Mushrooms are one of the oddest: Their toxins are only activated by alcohol (even a glass of wine within seventy-two hours is enough). Avoid picking wild mushrooms unless you are an expert, or accompanied by an expert, and be cautious when buying locally grown mushrooms such as at farmers' markets or roadside stands.

Deciding About Irradiated Produce

IRRADIATION OF OUR foods, including produce, is coming into wider use. Studies show that consumers worldwide are more accepting of it than they were ten or so years ago. But many of us are still uncomfortable with eating irradiated food. The general reaction of most people I know (including my own family) is that, given a choice, they would rather *not* eat it. Irradiation just sounds so unpleasant and unnatural. If the process were named "ionization" or something similar, it would sound less threatening. But does irradiation really make our food safer, and does the process itself make our food unhealthy? Well, about the only thing we can be absolutely sure of is that irradiated food is not radioactive, as some people fear.

Irradiation, or "ionizing radiation," is a process that briefly bombards food with high-frequency energy that damages the DNA of any bacteria, insects (such as fruit flies), or parasites in it. When low doses are used for fruit or vegetables, they can extend its shelf life by preventing sprouting and delaying ripening (important in our factory food system). At high doses, irradiation kills most bacteria and molds. At the medium-dose level that tends to be used for produce, irradiation does not kill all microbes in the fruit or vegetable or the toxins or spores they produce, but it will reduce their numbers and damage or inactivate *most* of them.

In August 2008, the U.S. government announced that it would also allow irradiation of some fresh produce, such as commercially produced spinach and iceberg lettuce. Irradiation was already in use for some other foods (such as herbs and spices, eggs, wheat flour, and meat and poultry) and was in limited use for some imported fruit. Canada also allows irradiation of such foods as onions, potatoes, wheat and whole wheat flour, and whole or ground spices and dehydrated seasonings. The argument for irradiating the spinach and lettuce was that this would kill or damage those *Salmonella, E. coli,* and other dangerous bacteria that have entered a spinach or lettuce leaf or that have developed tough bacterial communities that can't be washed off. Irradiation will probably inactivate or kill 95 to 99 percent of any organisms present, whereas washing well may only eradicate 90 to 95 percent.

How good or bad food irradiation is for our health remains controversial. The FDA, USDA, WHO, FAO—and, you will be relieved to know, the International Atomic Energy Agency—all reassure us that irradiation—if correctly done, of course—is no more dangerous than pasteurization or canning. So does the International Consultative Group on Food Irradiation (ICGFI), which was set up by the United Nations to study the issue. In fact, the report of the ICGFI basically blames consumers and the industry for being too conservative (read "technology troglodytes") in being reluctant to accept this wonderful scientific advance.

You will find arguments for using irradiated foods, including irradiated produce, in institutional settings, such as retirement and nursing homes, and schools. However, on the other side, critics of food irradiation say that it is not much use, and is simply a "cop-out"—it gives a false sense of security. That is, people using irradiated food are likely to skip other safety measures, thinking they are not needed. And we need to keep in mind that not only does irradiation not kill all microbes in the food, but irradiated food can become contaminated all over again. Irradiation only kills off what *was* in the food; it doesn't prevent it from picking up new germs. Critics also say that too little testing has been done on the safety and wholesomeness of irradiated foods—are the molecules of the foods themselves affected by it, as with genetic modification, and if so, what might that do to our body? What is more, there have been no long-term studies of how eating irradiated food will affect us over several decades.

Those strongly opposed to irradiation of food, such as the non-profit public interest group Public Citizen, argue that research dating to the 1950s has revealed a wide range of fairly horrible health problems in animals that ate irradiated foods. These critics and others have also pointed to the fact that irradiation can reduce vitamin levels and disrupt other nutrients in the food. Supporters of irradiation, such as ICGFI, say that this is no more so than in other forms of preservation such as drying, canning, and heat pasteurization. Then there is also another side to the issue. To the sensitive palate, irradiation can ruin the texture and flavor of some produce, as in the case of lettuce.

The food industry likes irradiation because it prevents some products such as potatoes and onions from sprouting; delays ripening in such produce as bananas, mangoes, and papaya; and helps delay spoilage in delicate fruits such as strawberries. Let's face it, it may also let them off the hook in case of an outbreak.

So where does that leave us? Basically, it leaves us waiting to see what may be revealed from long-term studies on the effects of eating irradiated food . . . and keeping our fingers crossed. Mind you, in the meantime, reading labels (see page 77) and eating organic produce can give you peace of mind if you are not too happy with the idea of irradiation.

Eating the Wax on Apples

REMEMBER THE OLD days when you could bite into an apple without getting a mouthful of tasteless wax? Unpleasant, yes, but is it harmful to our health?

Before being sent to the store, produce is sometimes extensively washed to clean off dirt, soil, and contaminants. This also removes the original oils and the protective natural wax coating that exists on many fruits and vegetables—such as apples, pears, plums, and watermelon—which repels water and also reduces water loss during storage. The wax that is added back by the industry does much the same thing. It helps to retain moisture during shipping, storage, and marketing, and reduces bruising. And it encourages us to buy the fruit. A nice shiny apple always looks better than a dull one, although the dull one often tastes a lot better.

The wax used by the food industry is considered to be harmless "natural" wax. The type of wax approved for the American food supply can come from plants, insects (such as bees), or food-grade petroleum products. It has to meet FDA Food Additive regulations.

We tend to think of commercial wax coating as being on fruit, but vegetables can have it, too. Look around next time you are in the produce section of your local grocery and just gently run your finger along the surface of some items on display. (It feels like touching a candle.) The kinds of produce you are likely to find with a wax coating include apples, cantaloupes, grapefruit, lemons, limes, oranges, passion fruit, peaches, and pineapples, as well as avocados, bell peppers, cucumbers, eggplant, parsnips, pumpkins, rutabagas, squash, sweet potatoes, tomatoes, turnips, and yuca.

Yes, organic fruits and vegetables may be waxed, too. Most organic produce is not, but some items may be, such as cucumbers, summer squash, and citrus fruit. The reasons for waxing organic produce are the same as those for conventional produce—to keep it fresh and attractive. You guessed it—not everyone who eats organically finds the thought of consuming an applied coating attractive. Besides, some kinds of wax simply don't sound as though they quite fit with organic principles.

Is this wax coating used on produce unhealthy? By the way, you won't be able to wash wax off, either, so there is no point even trying. But any waxes we eat on produce will not be digested. Wax passes through the body. The Produce Marketing Association (which is obviously biased) says that extensive research "by governmental and scientific authorities" has shown that the waxes we are presently eating in our food are perfectly safe. The government gurus agree. But there is little research on the issue.

But don't for a moment think that produce is the only waxed food we eat. Some chocolates and candy bars have added wax, too, which is why they turn white if put in the refrigerator. (Try it with some of your favorites.) Even many recipes for homemade chocolate-coated candy call for adding paraffin wax to melted dipping chocolate, for a smooth coating that adheres properly and makes the candy more stable as well. But let's face it, that wax-coated chocolate tastes a lot better than a wax-coated apple.

Cooking Potatoes with Less Acrylamide

THIS BOOK DOES not cover chemicals that are produced during cooking, a huge topic in itself (some eight hundred have been identified, perhaps fifty of which—particularly those relating to overheated oils and barbecued meats—are carcinogenic). There are other comprehensive books that you can read if you are interested in this subject (see appendix 4). However, I am making an exception in the case of one of the most recently identified and riskiest toxic compounds produced during cooking: acrylamide. I believe that in the next few years we will recognize this chemical as a major danger in our North American food supply.

Acrylamide is formed through something called the "Maillard reaction." It occurs when certain foods containing sugars and an amino acid are cooked at high temperatures. CDC testing has found that a large percentage of the U.S. population carry this potentially cancer-causing chemical in their body, in part because it is also present in cigarette smoke. At the same time, the United States has been slow to recognize acrylamide in food as being a health risk—much slower than the European countries, which years ago started to take action to reduce its levels and to educate the public.

One produce item that may be most to blame for our body burden of acrylamide could be a favorite: French fries and most potato chips (see sidebar). Some other produce items that have been found to contain high levels include prunes and some other dried fruit, prune juice, black olives, and asparagus. Everyone who eats cooked or processed food gets a bit of acrylamide in some way or another. But if you eat a lot of these foods, you may get more than is good for you. (See www.cspinet.org for levels in potatoes and other foods).

DON'T BURN THE FRENCH FRIES

It is believed that the average American eats some fifty-one pounds of French fries a year. Potatoes can carry a hefty load of acrylamide—as well as some other toxic substances. Although levels vary, French fries and pan-fried potatoes (as well as potato chips) tend to have much higher amounts of acrylamide than baked, boiled, or microwaved potatoes. But what if you really want those fried potatoes, or even worse, your children do?

The good news is that although we cannot completely remove acrylamide from our cooked foods, we can reduce its levels. This applies to fried potatoes, especially if we cook them ourselves.

Without guaranteeing that any of these measures work, here are some ideas from various countries that are struggling with the issue. First, don't store your potatoes in a cold refrigerator, which will make things worse when you cook them; keep them at room temperature. Second, you may want to first soak the potatoes for 15 to 30 minutes before cooking (the Germans say one hour), which helps to reduce the amount of acrylamide formed during cooking. Third, if you really must eat those French fries, make big fat ones (not the skinny fries). Fourth, make sure that they are golden brown but not dark brown. Brown areas are likely to contain more acrylamide. (Send them back if your children get darker brown ones in a restaurant, even if you don't worry about yourself.) Fifth, use oil with a high smoke point, such as corn oil, not olive oil (the Canadians say this step alone would generate 50 percent less acrylamide). Sixth, try boiling or microwaving the potatoes a bit first before you start to superheat them in oil. Finally, according to the Canadians, you may be able to reduce the levels by another

50 percent by adding rosemary—which also makes the potatoes taste better. According to the Finns, you can use a Finnish commercially produced flavonoid-based spice (which we can't advertise) to get the same effect. Some other additives that have been suggested are calcium chloride, citric acid, lactic acid, and phytate. Rosemary sounds about the best. Enzyme products that apparently help to reduce acrylamide have now come out in several countries.

Also, remember that other dishes such as Turkish *tulumba,* Norwegian *lefse* and *lompe,* Swiss *rosti,* and Spanish *neules* contain potatoes cooked at high temperatures.

Read Those Labels

THESE DAYS, WE have a variety of labels on our produce. Some are useful for making smart decisions to reduce our food risks. That is, if you know what they mean. The following may help.

Country of Origin Labeling (COOL)

Country of Origin Labeling (COOL) is a law that requires producers to provide their customers with country of origin information for those commodities that are covered by the law. Strictly speaking, COOL has more to do with our "right to know" than with safety, but the two *can* be related. In the United States, COOL was authorized by the 2002 and 2008 Farm Bills, and was implemented progressively in the food supply. COOL labeling allows us to make buying decisions based on where the food product comes from. We are now learning that this can be useful in helping us avoid foods from certain countries whose safety records we don't trust, or just helps us buy domestic if we wish. During the early stages of the 2008 *Salmonella* bacteria outbreak in fresh produce, when tomatoes from Mexico were (wrongly) suspected, we were advised to look for country-of-origin as a guide to safety.

Mandatory country-of-origin labeling for fresh produce went into effect in late 2008. It is being regulated by the USDA's Agriculture Marketing Service. More than half of produce in U.S. stores already carried such labeling prior to the deadline. However, although country-of-origin labeling is required for fresh fruits and vegetables, it is not for most processed produce such as frozen vegetable mixes or even for bagged salad mixes. As a result, most of our annual six billion pounds of imported processed produce (including canned peaches, mushrooms, and olives) will *not* have country-of-origin labels, at least as of time of writing.

Certified Organic

For any food product to be labeled and sold as "organic" in North America, it has to comply with national standards for organically produced commodities and be certified as "organic." For single-ingredient products such as fruit or vegetables, it is a black-and-white situation— they are either organic or "conventionally grown" (that is, non-organic). But both the United States and Canada require any multi-ingredient food that carries the organic label labeled to be at least 95 percent organic. In the United States, the National Organic Program (NOP), run by the USDA, outlines organic standards and generally oversees organic foods. In Canada, the CFIA is in charge.

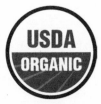

Figure 1

Organic farming systems for fruits and vegetables only use conventional pesticides as a last resort. (Most try not to use pesticides at all.) They rely instead on ecologically based pest control practices, such as cultural and biological pest management. Nor do organic producers use fertilizers made with synthetic ingredients or sewage sludge. Bioengineering or ionizing radiation are also out. Both domestic growers and those who supply our imported produce have to keep to these standards if they carry organic certification. But the labels will vary. Organic growers and organic handlers have to be certified by state or approved private agencies/organizations, under the government organic program standards. They can carry the government seal (see figure 1), another one, or both. There are some seventy-six approved organic certifying bodies in North America at the time of writing (fifty-five in the United States, twenty-two in Canada).

Very small farming operations are exempt from certification. Because of the complications of the certification process and the paperwork and expense involved, some slightly larger farms may not apply for certification, either, except in cases where they have a guaranteed market (such as a cooperative) that would make it worthwhile. However, this does not necessarily mean that such farming operations do not follow organic practices—maybe they are even better than some certified ones, though you will have to take their word for it. At the time of writing, major failings have been revealed in federal oversight of the organic food industry in the United States. For additional information, go to http://www.ams.usda.gov/AMSv1.0/nop.

Sustainably Farmed

Organic and sustainable farming share certain production principles, but they are not the same. Sustainable farming or sustainable agriculture is basically low-input farming, with an emphasis on resource conservation. It has a somewhat more flexible approach toward synthetic pesticides than does organic farming. But it uses only small amounts, relying as much as possible on other alternatives to control pests. Some organic production is not "sustainable," and some "sustainable farms" are not 100 percent organic. Sustainable farms tend to be small operations and sell their produce locally. But that is not *always* the case. There are no formalized standards for sustainable farming, but there is a shared broad and attractive philosophy.

Produce Dating

On fresh produce, as on other items, a "best if used by" date gives you the last date you should be eating this product if you want the best quality. Although this should not be considered a safety date, you may want to use it as a guide to freshness, as freshness does play a role in safety as well as nutritional benefits of fruits and vegetables.

PLU Codes

Sometimes one of the best ways to know how your produce is grown is to look at the tiny attached label with the PLU sticker and a four- or five-digit stock number. This is a particularly good idea if you want to avoid genetically modified produce (see sidebar), or want to make really sure that the fruits and vegetables in the so-called organic section are really organically produced. Most people I know never do this or know how to interpret the PLU sticker numbers. My spot checks suggest that many store managers won't be able to tell you what they mean, either. They just rely on their suppliers. Here is the key (same in Canada as in the United States):

A five-digit number beginning with 9 means the item has been organically grown.

A four-digit number beginning with 3 or 4 means that the item has been conventionally grown.

A five-digit number beginning with 8 means that the produce has been genetically modified (see sidebar).

THE ISSUE OF GENETICALLY MODIFIED FOOD

The topic of genetically modified (GM) food or genetically engineered (GE) food is huge and complex, far too large to cover adequately in this book.

Briefly put, GM food is here to stay. In the United States, in 2008, fully 80 percent of all corn and 92 percent of all soybeans grown were genetically modified varieties. GM companies are constantly developing new plant varieties. When farmers plant GM crops, they gain higher yields and reduce production costs. Scientists are also developing genetically engineered animals for a variety of purposes, one of them being more efficient food production. GM salmon may soon be available on the U.S. market, in spite of wide opposition. Increasingly, GM foods are everywhere, and difficult to avoid.

Both the U.S. and Canadian governments have basically taken the position that GM foods are "substantially similar" to other "normal" foods and will do us no harm. Government states that it will make sure that only GM animals or crops or fish that are "safe to eat" enter our food supply. We hope so.

But do we consumers really care? Yes, there have been a few instances (GM potatoes, wheat, and fish) where consumer organizations have bravely fought the powerful industry giants such as Monsanto. But most of us seem to have more or less forgotten about the GM issue (just as we seem to have done in the case of growth hormone use in food animals). Surveys show that the majority of us are also fairly ignorant about GM in general, and about the extent to which genetically modified organisms (GMOs) are in our food supply. Since they are not usually labeled, or we consumers do not know how to read labels (as in the case of PLU numbers on produce), most of us innocently consume GM foods without knowing we are doing it.

Yes, you could certainly argue for the positive potential of GMOs, such as helping to decrease world hunger (through the development of drought and disease-resistant varieties), increasing the nutritional value of foods (as in the case of adding vitamin A to rice or lysine to corn), and even in protecting the safety of our food (as could be the case if BSE-resistant cattle were developed). But at the same time, GMOs may be creating serious health and environmental risks that may not be able to be reversed. Some of the human and animal health-related concerns raised by organizations such as the Organic Consumers Association, the Union of Concerned Scientists, Friends of the Earth, and the American Council on Consumer Interests focus on the risks of food toxicity, allergens, antinutrients, and eventual contribution to antibiotic resistance. But wider agricultural, environmental, and health concerns exist as well. For instance, Greenpeace says that GM fish are a major threat to the world's oceans and could cause irreversible damage to wild fish.

Perhaps the biggest concern among many experts is that we still do not know what all the risks of GMOs are, and by the time we find out, it may be too late to do much about them.

Treated by Irradiation

Increasingly, American consumers can choose between irradiated and nonirradiated foods. If a product such as a fruit or vegetable is irradiated, the international symbol for irradiation, the "radura" (see figure 2) has to appear on the packaging, on bulk containers, or on a placard nearby

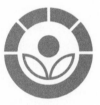

Figure 2

if the fresh produce is unpackaged. This symbol can be any color and be accompanied by a statement such as "treated by irradiation" or "with irradiation." Restaurants do not have to tell their customers if the produce they use has been irradiated; however, some voluntarily provide irradiation information on their menus.

Coated with Wax

U.S. federal law requires produce shippers and packers of waxed fruit or vegetables to state as much on the containers. Retailers are supposed to pass this information on to the public with a notice on the sales bin or counter. But good luck finding a sign in your store that says something like, "Coated with food-grade vegetable wax/paraffin/beeswax/shellac-based wax or resin, to maintain freshness." Most store managers seem to know nothing about it.

Warning on Juices

To protect consumers, unpasteurized juices now have to carry a warning label (see figure 3).

> WARNING:
> This product has not been pasteurized and therefore may contain harmful bacteria that can cause serious illness in children, the elderly, and persons with weakened immune systems.

Figure 3

But What About . . . ?

If I avoid spoiled-looking fruits and vegetables, will I be safe from microbes such as bacteria?

No, not necessarily. True, damaged fruit is more likely to also carry bad microbes. But fruit or vegetables can look perfectly good but still be contaminated. Many contaminants do not make produce look "spoiled." All the same, it is better to avoid buying fruit with a broken skin or a noticeable bruise. If you have a partly spoiled fruit or vegetable, throw the spoiled part out, particularly if it is soft fruit. If you belong to a high-risk group, you would be wise to toss the entire item.

Should I wash packaged produce labeled "prewashed"?

The FDA recommends washing raw produce repeatedly under running water (assuming you don't have water rationing) and scrubbing any tough surface of a fruit or vegetable (such as the skin of a potato). The experts go back and forth as to whether rewashing the packaged produce items that are labeled "prewashed" will further help to remove pesticides and microbes. There is little proof that it helps a lot. But it doesn't hurt, either, if you consider that microbes could have been multiplying beneath that plastic.

Do I need to wash organic produce from my own garden?

Yes, definitely. Organic produce also needs to be washed. That includes fruits and vegetables from your own garden or patio pots and even fruit that you grow on your own trees. In spite of all your care, they may still have been contaminated by insects, migrating birds, or wild animals. Every time I look at those squirrels that are constantly checking—and eating—the figs, plums, guava, and apples in my garden, I know they could be carrying anything. So could those raccoons and deer that attack my grapes and corn. As for all those birds I love having there . . .

Will refrigeration kill dangerous microorganisms?

You should not rely on refrigeration for killing microbes. Viruses and parasites survive the cold well. But bacteria— except for *Listeria monocytogenes,* which is especially dangerous for pregnant women—may not multiply as fast while refrigerated, so it makes sense to refrigerate ripe produce.

Do retailers wash produce before selling it?

Usually supermarkets and other produce retailers do not wash produce before putting it out because it has usually already been washed before it arrives at the store. However, many stores mist produce while it is on display so that it stays fresh looking. As long as the water used is clean, this will do no harm and may even drain away some remaining residues of those pesticides that dissolve in water.

Smart Ways to Reduce Your Risks

"HEALTHY" FRUITS AND vegetables may not be nearly as healthy as we think—even organic and locally grown ones. But you can limit your risks and still enjoy their health benefits by making smart decisions. If you want to avoid all the frustration (and mind you, a lot of pleasure) involved with gardening, there are some other things you can do to be safer. If you have a high-risk rating, you need to be particularly careful.

. . .

Use best practice when growing or collecting your own produce. Keep domestic animals away from ground-level produce, and keep an eye on wildlife, as both can carry contaminants. Water with clean water (look for eco-hoses that are safe to drink from if you wish to be extra careful). Organic practices are still best, although they are likely to leave you struggling with the bugs and with a somewhat reduced harvest. Pick your fruit or vegetables just before eating. Collect wild mushrooms only if you are an expert or accompanied by an expert.

Buy whole, healthy produce. Buy healthy-looking, firm fruits and vegetables without damaged areas, bruising, or broken skin, which could allow easier entry of contaminants. (Feel and smell the fruit, even if people stare at you!) If you are shopping in stores, read the labels (see pages 77–83) for country of origin and PLU sticker numbers, and look out for the irradiation radura if trying to avoid irradiated fruits and vegetables. Fruit with attached vines or stems, as in the case of tomatoes or strawberries, tend to be safer. Don't leave the produce sitting in your warm car any longer than you have to, particularly if it is in closed plastic bags.

Avoid RTE products whenever possible. Especially shun those in which different kinds of produce are mixed in together. RTE products are more likely to carry microbes of human origin. If you insist on buying fresh-cut produce (such as slices of melon) or bagged salad greens, make sure they have been kept on ice or in a refrigerator at the store or market.

Buy domestic and organic if you can. Generally, you are safer with domestic rather than imported produce, for avoiding both toxic pesticide residues and certain microbes. Farmers' markets, community-supported farms, organic cooperatives, and local produce vendors are great places to buy, but that may not always be possible. Check your local supermarket: More and more are beginning to carry organic goods, sometimes among conventional products rather than in their own special section; read the signs and PLU stickers. Buying organic produce will help you reduce your exposure to pesticide residues, avoid irradiation (if you don't want it), and sometimes avoid wax, but will not protect you against microbes or natural toxins. You can help your food budget by being selective about your organic produce (see page 66).

Store correctly. If the fruits and vegetables you buy are ripe, eat them as soon as possible to get best nutrition value and reduce chances of spoilage and waste. If you need to keep them for a while, then store as directed in the sidebar, checking frequently for moisture and spoilage. How long you can safely keep different fruits and vegetables will vary from a day to several weeks. Examples of ones you should usually eat in one to three days if stored in the refrigerator are: berries, broccoli, and corn, and any tomatoes stored at room temperature. Those that will usually last up to five to seven days if refrigerated properly include: spinach, summer squash, ripe tomatoes, and bell peppers. At room temperature, bananas and avocados usually fall into that group, but it depends how ripe they are when purchased. Produce that can last for a week or even more in the refrigerator include: lettuce and carrots (if stored separate from fruits), avocados, and apples. And at room temperature, onions and garlic (if stored away from potatoes), potatoes, oranges, and lemons. Winter squash can last for months.

SMART STORAGE OF FRESH FRUITS AND VEGETABLES

◇ **Store at room temperature, in a dry, cool place, out of the sun:** bananas (until ripe), tomatoes (unless very ripe) avocados, garlic, lemons, mangoes, onions, oranges, and potatoes. Oranges and lemons can also be stored in the refrigerator. Some also advise keeping carrots, parsnips, and peppers at room temperature.

◇ **Store in the refrigerator crisper, usually in an open or perforated plastic bag (set your refrigerator at 40°F or below):** apples, asparagus, bell peppers, berries, broccoli, carrots, celery, lettuce, peaches, peas, plums, spinach, ripe tomatoes, and others.

◇ **Store separately:** Store onions away from potatoes (as potatoes give off moisture), and fruit away from vegetables such as lettuce. Some fruit such as apples, avocados, bananas, cantaloupes and honeydew melons, peaches, pears, plums, and tomatoes give off ethylene gas, which encourages spoilage and "off" flavors in certain vegetables. Bitter-tasting carrots are an example of the effects of this gas.

◇ **Do spot checks:** Throw out any fruit or vegetable showing signs of spoilage or that smell bad, as spoilage will spread quickly to others. Remove moisture if it accumulates in the crisper or storage containers.

Wash, wash, wash. The goal of washing produce is to remove any remaining soil, chemical residues, and harmful organisms such as bacteria and parasites. True, it may only work 95 percent or so of the time, particularly if microbes have entered the flesh of the fruit or vegetable. But it is better to have two hundred organisms than four thousand. The FDA recommends washing under running water or rinsing multiple times, and tells us to scrub tough-skinned vegetables such as potatoes. Detergents or chemicals are not usually advised, as they are unhealthy. If you feel better doing it, make a solution of vinegar and water; of vinegar, salt, and water; or of vinegar, lemon juice, and water for rinsing purposes. Wash this off with plain water afterward, as skins of fruits and vegetables can absorb the flavor. Proportions recommended vary, but try 2 to 4 tablespoons of salt, the juice of a lemon, and 4 tablespoons of white vinegar to about three times as much clean water (you can omit the lemon). Some recommendations are for a twenty-minute soak, whereas others are for a quick rinse, followed by a rinse with plain water afterward. Just don't waste your money on buying a commercial fruit wash. Scrub any hard peels. Some people recommend using a little baking soda to help remove wax. (I am always amazed at how many uses baking soda has.)

Do not wash before storage. But you may be coming home from the farmers' market with a beautiful bunch of organic carrots just pulled from the soil, which are heavily covered in dirt; in that case, you may need to break that rule. Just make sure you dry them well afterward before storage. Generally speaking, however, wash immediately before use.

Peel if you can. Peeling is a good way to get rid of hardy microbes on the surface that do not wash off, resistant chemical residues, wax, and some natural toxins that tend to accumulate at higher levels in the peel. Wash before peeling so that your knife does not carry any contaminants on the outside into the flesh of the fruit or vegetable. Remove the outer layer of items such as cabbage, head lettuce, and leeks.

Trim when needed. Cut off and throw away any parts of a *hard* fruit or vegetable that look rotten, moldy, or discolored (as in the case of small green areas on potatoes, which can have natural toxins), along with a good-size safety margin. If the moldy fruit or vegetable is soft (for instance, berries or peaches), or if the produce has many bad spots (or, in the case of potatoes, the majority of the skin has a green tinge) it is better to discard the whole item, as parts of the mold or other contaminant may be invisible, and toxins can travel. Do the paring or discarding gently so that spores do not fly off and contaminate your kitchen environment or trigger your allergies.

Always pay attention to contamination risks. Ideally fruit or vegetables should be prepared just before they are to be cooked or eaten (that is, not leaving them around in a cut-up or "wounded" state to collect microbes). If necessary, refrigerate immediately after preparation. And remember to use good hygiene when preparing produce—avoid cross-contamination with other foods, especially raw meat and poultry, fish, or products that contain them. Wash preparation tools such as knives and boards, and your hands frequently. If you think you may have had a virus infection (such as the very contagious norovirus), do not prepare food for about three days afterward. Look at it as a good chance to have a rest.

Keep your kitchen clean. Obviously, a clean kitchen is important for all food safety. However, remember that some viruses are even resistant to detergent sprays, so it is best to make sure you don't contaminate counters or your sink (and faucet handles) in the first place. Clean ovens (including microwaves) of drips and spatters that could develop microbes. If you notice mold in your refrigerator or other appliances, or in a bin where you have stored produce at room temperature, it is best to wash it thoroughly with a bleach solution, or you will soon find other foods becoming moldy. Use a dedicated cutting board for produce, separate from any board you use for meats or poultry, as both wooden and plastic cutting boards can absorb microbes. Most important, wash cutting boards well, and throw them out if they become heavily scarred or discolored by mold.

Use cooking to reduce risks. Cooking is still a good way to reduce microbe risks, including in produce. Most of us will keep eating a lot of raw fruits and vegetables, but those with high food-risk ratings may want to seriously think about cooking to inactivate bacteria, parasites, and viruses (sorry, raw foodies). But how you cook is also important, not only for retaining nutrients, but also for avoiding **cooking chemicals** such as acrylamide.

Avoid risky juices. Packaged raw (unpasteurized) juices and ciders pose more safety risks than pasteurized juice. Vulnerable people, in particular, should avoid them. It is best to make your own, so that you can have both the health and the safety benefit, or to eat the whole fruit or vegetables instead. If you like to use juice bars, watch how the juice is made and ask questions (for example, "Are the carrots organic, washed, and peeled?") and use your judgment.

Eat out with care. Avoid raw vegetables, sliced fruit, freshly made salsa, guacamole, and fresh fruit salads, except in restaurants that you are sure procure the best produce and practice good hygiene. Also avoid eating these foods at catered affairs or in institutional settings. From a safety point of view, salad bars are best avoided for two reasons: the food is extensively handled, and it tends to sit out for a long time in not-the-best conditions.

Avoid raw produce when traveling to riskier countries. Especially avoid anything that grows close to the ground. If you are really dying for something raw, select something like a banana or mango and eat whole fruit only after you carefully wash and peel it, not fruit that has been sliced by someone else.

5

Fish and Shellfish

"**E**AT FISH, LIVE longer. Eat oysters, love longer." Whoever said that was only partly right. When raw, oysters are one of the most dangerous foods you could eat.

Whether fish extends your life span—or shortens it—depends on which fish you eat, how you eat it, and how much. We've all been told that fish is good for us. It is a great source of low-fat proteins and good nutrients, including omega-3 fatty acids, vitamins A and D, as well as trace elements such as selenium, zinc, fluoride, and iodine. Eating fish helps to prevent heart disease and is also important for a healthy brain, bones, nervous system, and eyes. Fish is also low in fat. What more could you want in a food? The American Heart Association recommends that you eat fish regularly—once or twice a week, or even more.

A few decades ago, fish used to be considered one of the safest foods you could eat. That is no longer the case. These days, seafood may well be the riskiest food you can eat. It's not if you count the number of illnesses (produce wins for that category), but it is if you define risk by the number of outbreaks caused in our food supply (although most are small), or if you think in terms of possible longer-term damage to your health. Shellfish is particularly high-risk.

Eating seafood can become a trade-off between nutrition and safety—just as it is can be with produce.

What We Eat

LET'S LOOK AT the seafood we eat. People in countries such as Iceland, Finland, Norway, and Sweden eat much more fish and shellfish than we do. Americans eat about sixteen pounds per person per year (some estimates put this as low as eleven pounds), with more of it eaten by higher-income households and in the Northeast than elsewhere in the country. Canadians eat more—about twenty-one pounds. There has been a general upward trend in the amount of fish and shellfish we eat. But some households eat none, whereas others eat it every week, and some even every day.

Roughly two thirds of the billions of dollars we spend every year on seafood is spent on meals in restaurants. Why not cook more seafood at home? Maybe it is partly that lingering, not-so-pleasant smell of fish in the house. Or is it simply that many people don't realize how quick and easy it is to prepare a delicious seafood lunch or dinner—or even a breakfast (salmon or trout and eggs can be a great change).

Our seafood-eating habits have changed over the last three decades. Instead of eating so much of it in tinned or cured form, as we used to, we are now eating more fresh and prefrozen seafood, increasing our safety risks. Only about a third of our fish and shellfish now comes in cans, much of it as tinned tuna.

More than 80 percent of the seafood eaten in the United States these days is imported—up from 55 percent in 1995—with well over half of it coming from Asia. All kinds of seafood are imported, including shrimp, tuna, salmon, groundfish, freshwater fish, crab, and squid. Our imported seafood is usually in frozen form, but we are likely to buy much of it "previously frozen."

The *kind* of fish and shellfish we like has not changed very much. According to the National Marine Fisheries Service, our favorite seafood (measured in pounds) is shrimp. Canned tuna is next in popularity. Other favorites are salmon, pollack, tilapia, catfish, crab, cod, clams, and flatfish (which in 2007 bumped out scallops). But in the future we may be eating less of our favorites, as ocean stocks are overfished and consumers become increasingly concerned about both environmental and safety issues in aquaculture.

THAT DELICIOUS, RISKY SHRIMP

If you live in the United States, you live in the country that eats the most shrimp in the world. Americans eat more shrimp than any other seafood. The National Fisheries Institute (NFI) estimates that, on average, this amounts to a little over four pounds of shrimp a year—down a bit from 2006. There are such wonderful shrimp dishes—shrimp scampi, shrimp pasta, shrimp cocktail, shrimp salad, grilled shrimp, garlic shrimp, Southern-fried shrimp, and Cajun shrimp, to name a few. You can keep shrimp in the freezer and drag it out for a last-minute meal that most people will enjoy. If someone tells you that they don't eat seafood, they often turn out to still eat shrimp. There are some twenty species of shrimp on the U.S. market. But if you love shrimp, you may not want to think about how some of them are raised.

Almost 90 percent of the shrimp eaten in the United States is imported and farm-raised. Almost half of the farmed shrimp, either Pacific whites or black tiger shrimp, comes from such countries as Thailand, Indonesia, Ecuador, China, Vietnam, Mexico, India, and Malaysia (in that order in 2009). How safe is this imported shrimp? No one really knows. With the few resources it has, the FDA does its best (which isn't much) to catch any shrimp that contains cancer-causing chemicals, drugs, or *Salmonella* or *Vibrio* bacteria before it arrives on our dinner plate. The FDA is also doing research on antibiotic-resistant bacteria in such shrimp, and the findings should certainly worry us (see page 111).

At least now, thanks to the 2009 federal COOL (Country of Origin Labeling) Act, all fresh and frozen seafood has to be labeled according to its source. That helps makes us aware of whether we are eating domestic or imported shrimp. Well, more or less. I checked out the choices I have in the three stores where I shop regularly (bringing along my magnifying glass). In one store, I found shrimp from China, Vietnam, and Thailand. In a second, shrimp from Indonesia. In the third, shrimp from Thailand. Where is *American* wild-caught or farmed shrimp?

Domestic shrimp is likely to be safer than imports, as how it is raised is more carefully controlled. At least in some parts of the United States, domestic fish farms are using environmentally friendly practices such as inland tanks. But domestic shrimp is usually also more expensive. And no one can guarantee that it will be completely free of contaminants, either. Our children's generation may find that they do not have a choice: domestic shrimp production is steadily decreasing, while imports are rapidly increasing. As for wild-caught (trap-caught) shrimp—they are much more expensive and hard to find even in Alaska and California. Just try locating them absolutely fresh (not frozen on board the vessel). Only a few top restaurants serve wild-caught shrimp—when they have it.

Seafood Is Becoming a High-Risk Food

IF WE ARE unlucky enough to become suddenly ill from eating seafood, the chances are that we caught a bad bacteria, parasite, virus, or a dose of a natural fish toxin. In addition, eating seafood can expose us to longer-term risk because of the unhealthy drugs, toxic chemicals, and heavy metals that much of farmed seafood carries these days. Knowing which seafood to eat is made still more complicated by the constantly changing safety advice to consumers and the increasing prices of some of our best fish. Add to this our concerns about depleting ocean stocks on one hand, and our worries about fish farming polluting the environment on the other. Why can't our decisions be simple—just based on what appeals to us?

The fact that our seafood is becoming more dangerous to eat has a lot to do with the fact we are eating more farmed seafood, especially more *imported* farmed seafood. Over 40 percent of the fish and shellfish that the United States imports is *farmed seafood,* and of this, about half comes from Asia—especially China, Vietnam, and Thailand. Over the last decade, China's exports of seafood to us have more than doubled.

Our scientists, regulators, and even politicians are increasingly recognizing that much of the farmed seafood we are getting from such countries as China and Vietnam may be produced and processed under conditions that are not up to U.S. standards. The existing safety gaps could pose health risks to you and me when we eat fish.

EATING SEAFOOD "MADE IN CHINA"

More and more of the fish and shellfish we eat is farmed in China. Is it safe to eat? America is not the only country worried about Chinese seafood. So are the European Union and other Asian countries such as Japan and Taiwan. There are good reasons to be concerned.

In the United States, a disproportionately high number of incoming shipments of seafood from China have been found to have safety violations. Most problems have been found in shrimp, catfish fillets, and eels. They have also occurred for such seafood as tilapia, tuna, monkfish, squid, crawfish, mackerel, crab, cod, and other popular species. Over the years, there has been a continuing pattern of seafood-related violations by China, with no sign of improvement.

The reasons FDA inspectors have given for rejecting shipments of Chinese seafood fall under the agency's usual broad categories, such as "too filthy for human consumption" (meaning that it has visible insects, dirt, human hairs, and so on), "unsafe additives" (such as colorants), "veterinary drug residues," "pesticide residues," "pathogens" (such as *Salmonella* and *Listeria* bacteria), or it has labeling problems. I noticed that heavy metals and **industrial chemicals** have also been found. In other words, you could say that just about everything nasty and unpleasant that could possibly turn up, *is* turning up in Chinese seafood shipments. FDA inspections at our ports are only catching a small fraction of these risky imported foods. Are you still planning to have fish for dinner?

In the case of Chinese farmed seafood, many of the problems are entering at the fish-farm level. Overcrowded conditions and high levels of pollution on fish farms result in constant health problems for the fish. Because no one wants to buy fish with horrible skin diseases and deformities, this has led Chinese fish farmers to use large doses of antibiotics, fungicides, and other pesticides—including some that are banned in the United States and Canada. Residues of these substances are turning up in our fish. When I was working on Chinese aquaculture, I noticed that some Chinese fish farmers who were told to use such nontraditional fish-farming practices refused to eat their own farmed fish!

So where does this leave us? Should we eat fish because it is good for us, or avoid it because it can ruin our health? The good news is that you can continue to eat fish and shellfish regularly, and feed it to your children and your elderly mother (and particularly, your mother-in-law), as long as you know how to make smart decisions about which seafood to eat and how to cook and eat it.

I would argue that being a smart and informed consumer is more important in the case of seafood than as regards any other food we eat.

Who Keeps It Safe?

KEEPING OUR FISH and shellfish safe is an increasingly important and difficult task. It has been estimated that some 130 countries are now exporting seafood to the United States, with about fifteen thousand registered foreign firms linking up to some three thousand U.S. importers. In addition, some thirteen thousand U.S. seafood processing establishments take it from there. We have a very complex seafood supply system. Add to this the problem of many different kinds of safety risks. Yes, efforts to keep on top of all this *are* being made by both government and the industry. They are not enough.

On the government side, the FDA is in charge, with other federal and state agencies also involved. Oversight of both domestic and imported seafood falls far short of what is needed. The FDA has a three-pronged approach to regulating *imported* seafood products (all of them weak): inspections of foreign manufacturers, inspections of U.S. importers, and inspection of entering shipments of seafood products. Sensibly, the FDA gives more of its attention to incoming shipments from countries that have a history of violations. But overall, the inspection rates of foreign firms that export seafood and the seafood they send to the United States have actually gone down, while imports have gone up. Only about 1.6 percent of incoming shipments of seafood are able to be inspected. This means that roughly nine hundred thousand shipments of seafood come in without even a "look-see." When inspections of seafood processing facilities here or overseas do occur, testing samples are taken in only a very small percentage of cases. Even in the case of seafood entering our ports, tests are only performed on about half of the *inspected* shipments (about 0.8 percent of all incoming shipments).

While the rate of FDA inspection and testing of seafood is actually higher than for other imported foods it oversees, it is *much* lower than we need for safety. Our rate of seafood inspection is also lower than that of most other industrialized countries that rely heavily on seafood imports.

Both the FDA and states agencies try to provide safety education for consumers through various kinds of advisories concerning the sources of domestic fish. State fish advisories alert us to the potential health risks of eating contaminated fish caught in state lakes, rivers, and coastal waters (but I constantly see people fishing such waters despite an advisory, and many of them probably eat the fish they catch). The EPA maintains a centralized database. The FDA as well as the state agencies also inform consumers about the safety risks in fish they buy. (Do you read them?) These are periodically updated when new research data on risk factors becomes available or our waterways become more polluted. Or when the experts simply change their mind.

Safety issues in seafood and advice to consumers are often hotly debated between the various government agencies, and between the FDA and industry organizations. The ongoing mercury debate and the 2009 controversy about the treatment of oysters (see page 103) are examples of such disagreements. In the final analysis, it currently seems that what is considered to be safe in our seafood is at least partly a matter of opinion, partly a matter of profit and politics, and only partly a matter of public health.

Avoiding All Those Parasites

DISEASE-CAUSING ORGANISMS such as parasites, bacteria, and viruses are hiding in our raw fish and shellfish more often than we realize. Marine mammals, particularly those delightful seals and sea lions in the northern Pacific and Atlantic oceans, can be involved. Such mammals often play a key role in the fish parasites' life cycle through excreting parasite eggs. Fish can get parasites from the infected crustaceans they eat (helped by the fact that they are the slowest and therefore easiest to catch) or from the smaller fish they consume.

Certain types of fish are higher risk for parasite larvae. It seems that our favorite wild-caught salmon, so healthy in other ways, is close to the top of that list. I found some statistics that said that 75 to 100 percent of all wild-caught Pacific salmon have been found to carry *Anisakis* spp. parasites (including sockeye, coho, and king salmon). Parasites are also fairly common in Atlantic salmon, not only in the intestinal cavity but also in the muscle. However, research has found that farmed salmon, if fed normal pelleted feed, have none. That situation changes if they are fed raw fish.

Both our marine and freshwater fish can actually carry the larvae or cysts of some very large parasites, such as roundworms and tapeworms. Some tapeworms are as much as forty feet long, can live twenty years, and produce a million eggs a day! They can be present not only in the gut of the fish but also in the flesh. Once the larvae are in *our* body, they can turn into the adult worm. Two common roundworms are the "cod worm" found not only in cod, but many other fish species as well, and the "herring worm" (see sidebar). North American fish that are likely to carry roundworms include rockfish, herring, mackerel, cod, whiting, and salmon. You could get tapeworms from freshwater fish such as trout and pike. Trematodes or flukes (flatworms) are also increasingly found in the freshwater fish and shellfish that we eat.

It is believed that one reason for the increase in such parasites is the fact that we are now getting more of our seafood from countries where fish may be farmed in unhygienic fishponds. Parasites can be present not only in fish but also in undercooked or cold-smoked octopus, squid, snails, and crabs/crayfish. If you do happen to eat a live parasite larva, you may be lucky. It could simply pass right through you without doing any harm. But if it doesn't, the results can be thoroughly unpleasant.

A WORM YOU DON'T WANT TO GET

As far as infectious worms go, *Anisakis simplex*—sometimes also called the "herring worm"—is pretty small and innocent looking. But it can be vicious. No one can convince you otherwise if you accidentally swallow this small roundworm in a mouthful of "healthy" raw fish. It is often found in herrings, mackerel, rockfish, whiting and blue whiting, but also in many other species of saltwater fish. The more you eat such uncooked dishes as sashimi, sushi, ceviche, or raw herring, the more likely you are to get an *Anisakis* bonus. Fish processors try to get rid of these parasites, but they miss some if they are well hidden in the fish tissues.

One of several things is likely to happen to you if you swallow this worm. The first—and most embarrassing, if you are dining with someone you want to impress—is that you feel an unpleasant tickle in your throat as the worm wriggles down. You gag and cough it up. Even if your dinner date never asks you out again, it is probably better than the alternatives.

If you do ingest the worm, let's hope it ends up in your stomach, intestine, or colon and decides to stay there for a while. True, in less than twelve hours the intense pain, cramps, and diarrhea will make you wish you were dead. You—and maybe your doctor—would probably think that you have Crohn's disease, appendicitis or an ulcer. But this can pass in a day or so, or at the most, seven to ten days, when the worm expires.

But this pesky parasite can also take up longer-term residence, as can occur if its larvae escape through the gastrointestinal wall and make lesions in your abdominal cavity, your pancreas, ovaries, uterus, liver, lung, or elsewhere in your body. In some instances, victims actually end up in surgery, believed to have a tumor. If this happens to you, the only upside is that you will be pleasantly surprised when the surgeon tells you that he (or she) just took out a round one-and-a-half-inch worm that had formed a granuloma (an inflamed mass of tissue). Maybe a piece of your intestinal tract had to go as well. But look on the bright side—no tumor.

So, if you end up in the emergency room soon after eating raw fish, you had better make a full confession to the attending doctor, even if he gives you a lecture. At least he will consider the possibility of anisakiasis before he tries to remove your appendix.

One fairly reliable rule you may want to remember is that in general, larger fish of the same species are more likely to carry a heavy load of parasites than are the smaller and younger fish.

There are two reasons: They eat more, therefore also ingesting a larger number of parasites, and parasite larvae can survive for a long time and build up in the body of fish as they get older.

Most parasites in your fish will be removed by gutting and cleaning. But any that have entered the flesh of the fish will be missed.

Seafood dishes vary in terms of risk. As with fruits and vegetables, you should put any raw or undercooked seafood dish at the top of your high-risk list—for example Italian *crudo*, South American ceviche, Japanese sushi and sashimi, and Scandinavian gravlax or lightly marinated herring. The good news is that fish parasites are killed by thorough cooking. The other good news is that there is a freezing technique that works, even for raw seafood dishes, if done right. The third bit of good news is that you shouldn't worry about eating a cooked or commercially frozen parasite larvae. You are unlikely to taste the worm. The chances are, you won't even know it is there.

Experts also believe that a large percentage of parasitic infections that originate in fish are never correctly identified—as is also the case with parasites in raw fruits and vegetables. The smart approach is to make sure you use the correct "kill step" for any parasite larvae in your seafood. To sum it all up:

What usually works:
- Cooking the fish thoroughly to an internal temperature of 145°F. Normal cooking procedures generally exceed this temperature.
- Smoking the fish at temperatures of 150°F.
- Commercial freezing of fish destined for raw fish dishes. The FDA recommends seven days at −10°F or fifteen hours at −31°F. Other recommendations are for −4° or −5°F for a minimum of five to seven days (or even as little as sixty hours).
- Irradiating seafood at sufficient levels. This usually either kills the larvae or prevents their developing into adults.

What cannot be relied on:

- Cleaning (gutting) and washing the fish. Although this will remove *most* parasite larvae, it will not work 100 percent.
- Salting or marinating the fish (salting with a 21 percent solution for ten days—some say five to seven days—would probably work, but who is going to do that?)
- Cold smoking such as kippering (which does not reach commercial smoking temperatures)

Evading Bacteria and Viruses

YOU CAN ALSO pick up disease-causing bacteria or viruses from seafood, particularly from certain types of fish or shellfish. Those that live in polluted waters are most likely to carry them. That is what makes molluscan shellfish—the two-shelled type, such as oysters, mussels, clams, and whole scallops—so dangerous. Mollusks like to live where rivers and seas meet, which is frequently where cities are located, with sewage contaminating the waters. Mollusks pump these filthy waters through their gills (an oyster can filter up to one hundred gallons of water a day!). In the process of getting the tiny organisms they want, they also pick up and store bacteria (such as *Salmonella*, *Shigella*, and *Vibrio*), viruses (such as norovirus), and other toxic substances. Our own preferences for eating them raw or lightly cooked adds to our risks. Raw oysters are the most dangerous shellfish we eat in terms of microbe risks, particularly for *Vibrio* bacteria and norovirus.

THE MOST DANGEROUS SHELLFISH

Oysters taste delicious and are low in mercury, but they are still the most dangerous kind of shellfish—particularly if eaten raw. Each year, there are many U.S. outbreaks of food poisoning linked to oysters. A few of these outbreaks have caused hundreds of illnesses, even though only a small fraction of Americans eat oysters at all.

The majority of oyster-associated illnesses are caused either by a norovirus or bacteria from the *Vibrio* genus (whose members includes the cholera bacterium). Symptoms of *Vibrio* infection appear within four hours to four days of **ingestion**. A *Vibrio* illness is likely to be much more dangerous than a norovirus-caused one. Most cases are not reported.

Vibrio bacteria are very common in brackish saltwater around the United States and in Canada, particularly during the summer. They are at some of their highest levels in Gulf of Mexico, and are often present in oysters and other shellfish harvested in the states of Florida, Texas, Louisiana, and Mississippi. Before the disastrous oil spill of 2010, this region supplied more than half of U.S. oysters.

People at greatest risk are those with liver disorders such as cirrhosis, hepatitis, and liver cancer; those whose immune systems are not functioning normally, as in the case of people with AIDS or cancer, or who are undergoing related treatments; those who have had gastric surgery or take a large amount of antacids; and those with kidney disease, diabetes mellitus, or hemachromatosis. Some *Vibrio* species are particularly vicious. The effects can be frightening and include not just fever, chills, confusion, diarrhea, but even occasionally loss of skin, kidney failure, and excruciating pain. Healthy people (such as my oyster-eating husband) have few problems with this shellfish. But about half of the high-risk people who become ill with the most dangerous *Vibrio* bacteria may die. No oyster is worth your life—even if it has a pearl in it.

In 2009, the FDA proposed that all oysters harvested from the Gulf states from April to October be required to undergo processing to kill *Vibrio* bacteria, effective summer of 2011. This was based on the California initiative of 2003, which considerably reduced oyster–related illnesses. However, after strong objections from Gulf Coast oyster harvesters (motivated by added costs), state officials (probably motivated by the oyster farmers and the thought of extra work), elected representatives (motivated by votes), and oyster purists (motivated by feared changes in flavor), the FDA backtracked. It suggested the usual—undertaking further consultations and

> more studies. So, in the meantime, you are on your own. You may just want to stick to well-cooked oysters or canned smoked oysters, if you love them.

Mollusks are not the only fish or shellfish that can carry bacteria and viruses. Nor are all contaminants there from the start. Seafood, like any other food, can also be contaminated by food handlers, equipment, and in other ways, *after* it is caught, and even after it is cooked. In fact, any seafood can carry microbes.

Some of the microbes you are likely to find in seafood, often entering at later stages, are "the usual culprits"—bacteria such as *Staphylococcus* and *Salmonella* and the hepatitis A virus (which infects the liver). At times the deadly Shiga-like toxin–producing *E. coli* and *Listeria* bacteria have also turned up. *Listeria* is most commonly associated with RTE seafood products (as it also is with RTE meats—see page 139, and dairy—see page 185). At the time I first wrote this, the FDA had posted product recalls in a period of a few months for such items as cooked langoustines from Chile, mussel meat from New Zealand, and tuna salad and deli tuna sandwiches, all because of possible *Listeria* contamination.

Sushi, unfortunately, tends to be a particularly risky dish and can give you a wide choice of bacteria (see sidebar).

SUSHI—HEALTH FOOD OR RUSSIAN ROULETTE?

The first American sushi bar opened in Los Angeles in 1964. Sushi soon caught on with businessmen and Hollywood celebrities. Now it is everywhere. Millions of Americans think that sushi is the guiltless, healthy fast food—the one they can eat three or four times a week, and teach their children to love. But is it?

Some researchers and nutritionists contend that sushi is anything but healthy. The rice part of it may be fairly harmless. But the other ingredients may contain parasites, dangerous bacteria, toxic chemicals, heavy metals, and pesticides. So what? Is it worse than any other food?

In some ways, yes, because many popular sushi dishes use raw fish. Eating raw seafood is always riskier than eating seafood that has been properly cooked. If you do eat sushi containing raw fish, you will be less likely to get a nasty parasite if the sushi is made in a restaurant that follows FDA guidelines to superfreeze the fish (including salmon, but not certain kinds of tuna). But that still does not protect you from many bacteria or viruses in the fish. They could be there to begin with, enter during the preparation process if good hygiene is not used, or multiply while the sushi is sitting around waiting for you in an unrefrigerated or poorly chilled display counter or mobile sushi track. Again, not all foods at the sushi bar are raw. But even those that are not may be carrying a heavy germ load, as a result of cross-contamination.

In recent years, several outbreaks of *E. coli, Salmonella, Listeria monocytogenes,* norovirus, and *Staphylococcus aureus* bacteria have been traced to sushi in various parts of the United States. One sizeable outbreak occurred in 2006 in Bentonville, Arkansas, when more than one hundred people became ill after eating at a local sushi restaurant. The culprit, apparently, was *Salmonella* bacteria. Bacteria and parasites in your sushi can give you some very unpleasant days (and nights) battling diarrhea, nausea, vomiting, and stomach cramps. Also, toxic substances such as mercury can expose you or your children to worse dangers over the longer term.

Keeping an Eye on Your Mercury Levels

A NUMBER OF toxic heavy metals are normally present in the earth. We pick up tiny amounts every day—through our skin, from air and water—and sometimes from our food. No problem—our body can deal with them. But if we pick up a bit too much of one of the more toxic metals over the years and it **bioaccumulates** (builds up in our body faster than we can metabolize or excrete it), we could be in trouble. It could affect our liver, kidneys, or circulatory or nervous system. Some heavy metals are potentially carcinogenic. Some have also been linked to birth defects.

Such metals as mercury, cadmium, lead, thallium, and arsenic can be present in waterways where fish and shellfish live. These metals get there through industrial pollution, waste, and even from the soil. There may be even higher levels in fish that is imported from countries where environmental controls are weaker and they are accumulating in the waterways (see sidebar, page 17). Yes, some of these toxic fish turn up during the inspection of incoming shipments, but many more get through.

In our seafood, one of the most important among such metals is the global pollutant methyl mercury. It is one of the biggest risks in seafood eaten in North America. Mercury is everywhere in our streams and oceans. FDA testing has found mercury to be present in *every* waterway in forty-seven states of America and in the tissues of fish from those waterways. When mercury levels are very high in freshwater lakes, rivers, or coastal waters, states will issue fish advisories. The number of states that have done so has risen steadily over the years. In New York State alone, some eighty waterways have restricted advisories for fish consumption because of the high levels of mercury.

Methyl mercury is invisible, odorless, and over the long term, it can be toxic to the brain and nervous system. Fish build it up in their body and pass it on to us. Because mercury builds up in their *muscle* tissue (not the gut or fat), there is no way of avoiding it when you clean, cook, or eat the fish. (Yes, you read that right. Cooking the fish does not destroy this toxic compound.)

As with some other foods we eat, eating fish can become a matter of treading a fine line between safety and nutrition—between getting too much mercury and making sure our body gets enough of those wonderful omega-3 fatty acids that we need for a healthy heart. How we decide which and how much fish to eat will depend a lot on who we are. The most significant risk is for young children and pregnant women, as well as women who may become pregnant in a year or two. But all of us need to pay attention. Often it becomes a matter of trade-offs.

Fish and shellfish vary considerably in their mercury levels. As a general rule, the bigger predatory fish—such as tilefish, swordfish, shark, king mackerel, and certain types of tuna and orange roughy—have the highest level because they eat smaller fish, and the mercury has had time to build up in their body. The smaller fish, lower down on the food chain (and on the fashionable fish hierarchy) are usually safer. These low-mercury risk fish include sardines, trout, herring, and pollack. They are also likely to be cheaper, which doesn't hurt.

Most of the popular seafood that is eaten in North America, such as shrimp, salmon, clams, catfish, scallops, pollack, cod flounder, and crabs, have comparatively low levels of mercury. That is, all except for our popular tuna—usually eaten in canned form (see sidebar).

LOVE THAT TUNA— BUT DON'T EAT TOO MUCH

Tuna is America's most popular fish. On the average, we eat almost three pounds per person per year—a little less than we used to. Many of us eat much more. Tuna (along with other fish such as swordfish, shark, and mackerel) get its mercury load from eating smaller fish that are contaminated with methyl mercury. Tuna tissues and body parts can have a concentration of mercury thousands of times higher than the mercury in its environment.

But different types of tuna vary because of their size and habitat. Bigeye, yellowfin, and albacore tuna are most likely to have higher concentrations of mercury—although Pacific troll-caught albacore has been found to have less. As a general rule, canned tuna labeled "light" has lower levels of mercury than does canned albacore because it uses mainly skipjack tuna. Exceptions have been found where yellowfin tuna has been mixed with the skipjack. The specific type of tuna used is not stated on the "light" tuna can. By the way, much of the canned tuna we eat these days is imported from Thailand.

> Tuna is, of course, popular not just in sandwiches and salads, but also as tuna steak and in sushi. *The New York Times* conducted an analysis of tuna sushi served in some of the better restaurants in New York (at the end of 2007, reported in January 2008). The report concluded that if you regularly ate six pieces of tuna sushi a week, your intake of mercury would exceed FDA-recommended safety levels. You might be at the greatest risk in an upscale restaurant, which is more likely to serve expensive bluefin tuna sushi—the tuna with the highest levels of mercury. In other words, high price does not mean low risk.

Although everyone agrees that methyl mercury can be dangerous, and that it is often present in fish, not everyone agrees on what that means in terms of safe fish eating. Even government agencies do not always agree. About the only thing that everyone does agree on is that methyl mercury risk is greatest for developing fetuses and young children. Let's look briefly at these two high-risk groups.

The still-developing nervous systems of young children are vulnerable to such substances as mercury. They may accumulate small amounts from several sources—apparently even from certain kinds of polyurethane flooring used in schools that, when damaged, can give off mercury vapors. That is all the more reason for making sure that our children's food is not adding mercury to what they get from those sources we can't control. Children younger than age six (some say even older) need to be the most careful. Because of the mercury risks involved, many experts and organizations, including the FDA, suggest that young children should eat no more than one small meal of albacore or white tuna a week. They can eat more "light" tuna. Probably a couple of "light" tuna sandwiches a week are safe. Other fish dishes that children may eat, such as fish sticks or fast-food fish sandwiches, are usually made with low-mercury fish, so they are not a concern.

Pregnant women have to be particularly careful about mercury in seafood. Excessive levels of it in the bloodstream of unborn babies have been associated with brain damage, mental retardation, poor coordination, blindness, seizures, autism, and developmental delays. Part of the problem is that mercury stays in the body for about eighteen months. This means that women who are trying to become pregnant should plan ahead. They should cut back seriously on their mercury uptake, to allow their body to eliminate it ahead of time.

The following classification of seafood is based on analyses and advice from a variety of sources, including the Natural Resource Defense Council (NRDC), the FDA, the American Pregnancy Association, the American Heart Association (Note: There are some differences of opinion).

- **Lowest mercury:** anchovies, butterfish, calamari (squid), catfish, caviar (farmed), clams, king crab, crawfish/crayfish, flounder or sole, haddock, hake, herring, rock lobster, oysters, ocean perch, pollack, salmon, sardines, scallops, shad, shrimp, sole, farmed sturgeon, tilapia, freshwater trout, whitefish
- **Low mercury:** carp, cod, blue crab, Dungeness crab, monkfish, freshwater perch, skate, snapper, snow crab, fresh Pacific albacore tuna, canned chunk "light" tuna
- **Higher mercury:** saltwater bass, bluefish, croaker, halibut, Maine lobster, mahimahi, sea trout, several varieties of tuna (canned white albacore, fresh bluefin, fresh ahi)
- **Highest mercury:** grouper, king mackerel, marlin, orange roughy, shark, swordfish, tilefish (golden bass or golden snapper)

Pregnant women need to remember that they can also get quite a lot of mercury from eating high-mercury sushi and similar foods. They can still eat it—but should choose carefully. If you love sushi, it would not be a bad idea to print out the following box, issued by the NRDC, and keep it in your wallet.

GUIDE TO MERCURY IN SUSHI

Lower-Mercury Fish

Akagai (ark shell)*
Anago (conger eel)*
Aoyagi (round clam)
Awabi (abalone)*
Ayu (sweetfish)
Ebi (shrimp)†
Hamaguri (clam)
Hamo (pike conger; sea eel)*
Hatahata (sandfish)
Himo (ark shell)*
Hokkigai (surf clam)
Hotategai (scallop)†
Ika (squid)
Ikura (salmon roe)
Kaibashira (shellfish)
Kani (crab)
Karei (flatfish)
Kohada (gizzard shad)
Masago (smelt egg)
Masu (trout)
Mirugai (surf clam)
Sake (salmon)
Sayori (halfbeak)*
Shako (mantis shrimp)
Tai (sea bream)*
Tairagai (razor-shell clam)*
Tako (octopus)

Tobikko (flying fish egg)
Torigai (cockle)
Tsubugai (shellfish)
Unagi (freshwater eel)*
Uni (sea urchin roe)

High-Mercury Fish

Ahi (yellowfin tuna)
Aji (horse mackerel)*
Buri (adult yellowtail)*
Hamachi (young yellowtail)*
Inada (very young yellowtail)*
Kanpachi (very young yellowtail)*
Katsuo (bonito)*
Kajiki (swordfish)†
Maguro (bigeye,† bluefin,† or
    yellowfin tuna)
Makjiki (blue marlin) †
Meji (young bigeye,† bluefin,† or
yellowfin tuna)
Saba (mackerel)
Sawara (Spanish mackerel)
Seigo (young sea bass)†
Shiro (albacore tuna)
Suzuki (sea bass)†
Toro (bigeye,† bluefin,†
    or yellowfin tuna)

*Mercury levels specific to these fish were not available and instead were extrapolated from fish with similar feeding patterns.
†Fish to avoid for other reasons than mercury, for instance, the fact that they are perilously low in numbers or are caught using environmentally destructive methods.

SOURCE: Natural Resources Defense Council: http://www.nrdc.org/health/effects/mercury/sushi.asp

Mercury is not the only toxic metal that can turn up in our seafood. Arsenic in fish? Yes, it happens. A few years ago the state of Utah issued an arsenic advisory for brown and cutthroat trout from the North Fork of American Fork Creek in Utah County. Pregnant women, nursing mothers, and children under age twelve were advised to avoid eating any trout from the creek. It was believed that the arsenic present was both natural and a result of mining contamination. Other metals such as cadmium, lead, and copper have also turned up in our seafood. The contaminated natural environment is not always the only source. I came across a case where the copper that was used to treat fish cages was believed to have been the cause of high levels of copper in farmed fish.

It may take decades to reduce the levels of mercury, arsenic, and such other potentially toxic metals in our own waterways. So don't expect the problem to go away anytime soon. Draft plans are in the works for reducing the mercury content of several key waterways in the United States. An example: In mid-July 2007, California adopted a cleanup plan for the San Francisco Bay—with a timetable of seventy years. The reason for the long timeline is the amount of mercury-laden sediment in the bay, not helped by the fact that an estimated 2,645 pounds of mercury are added to the bay's water each year from hundreds of sources.

We Don't Want Drug Residues in Our Farmed Fish

ANOTHER AREA FOR concern is drug residues in farmed seafood. Aquaculture in many of the countries from which we source our seafood uses huge amounts of drugs to combat the bacteria, viruses, molds, and parasites that thrive in the overcrowded food- and feces-filled fish farms. Diseases such as sea lice, skin and gill infections, and spotted fever spread rapidly from one fish to the next. Instead of reducing the fish density, the profit-focused industry prefers to load fish feed with large amounts of antibiotics, pesticides, and other chemicals. Farmed shrimp and salmon—two of our favorites—are among the seafood that may be given high levels of such substances. In open-water fish farms, where fish live in net pens, the surrounding waters become polluted with the uneaten drug-ridden food and floating drug-imbued fish waste. I was surprised to find that even some top aquaculture industry officials acknowledge the problem of dangerous drug overuse in fish farming. But that doesn't mean they are stopping it.

Testing over a period of four years has showed that seafood products imported to the United States from Asia (mainly the China, Vietnam, and Indonesia) and South American countries have been the worst offenders. Of the Asian countries, Vietnam and China showed the highest rates of drug-contaminated seafood. One year's testing of seafood shipments from Vietnam showed a contamination rate of 24 percent, and the next year those from China showed a 22 percent rate. Evidence has also been found of large Chilean salmon-farming operations using a number of dangerous pesticides and antibiotics not approved in the United States. Chile is the primary source of farmed salmon eaten in America.

Moreover, some of these substances are illegal. More shipments of shrimp are reported to be turned back at U.S. ports because of illegal drugs than are shipments of any other imported food. True, our overseas seafood farmers—as well as domestic ones—are only supposed to use those drugs that are on the FDA approved list. Also, they are only to be used according to FDA specifications that spell out which species they can be used for, dosage, method of administration, and withdrawal period. (The withdrawal period is meant to assure that no harmful drug residues will remain in the edible fish tissue when it is eaten.) But such regulations are often broken.

Several of the drugs that are turning up on testing of seafood imports are not approved in North America and are known or suspected carcinogens, or they are antibiotics that are now banned in the United States because of fear that they are encouraging **antibiotic resistance** in bacteria. Any incoming seafood shipment found to have illegal drug residues is not approved for import. The foreign manufacturers or shippers may also be placed on import alert. Sometimes an entire country is placed on such an alert, as happened in 2007 with China. But given the limited inspection and even more limited testing, how much is getting through to your local fish retailer?

Among the drugs that have been found to turn up in our imported farmed seafood are chloramphenicol (in shrimp and crabs); nitrofurans (in shrimp); fluoroquinolones (in bass, grouper, catfish, and tilapia); malachite green (in bass, eel, catfish, tilapia, salmon, and dace); quinolones (in salmon); and gentian violet (in catfish and shrimp).

DANGEROUS DRUGS THAT ARE TURNING UP IN OUR SEAFOOD

◇ **Fluoroquinolones:** A group of important broad-based antibiotics, also widely used for treatment of humans. The main risk posed by their use in fish farming is the increased development of resistance by bacteria. *An (ongoing) FDA study has found that our imported shrimp is already carrying numerous fluoroquinolone-resistant bacteria, including deadly ones such as* Vibrio *spp.,* Salmonella, *and* E. coli.

◇ **Nitrofurans:** A group of relatively inexpensive drugs, formerly widely used in food animal (and fish) production around the world. They are effective against many bacteria and fungi. Most nitrofurans are also mutagenic and carcinogenic. Their use in fish and food animal feed has been banned in the United States for years. Nitrofurans are still being manufactured, and many countries continue using them, including in fish farming.

◇ **Gentian violet (crystal violet) and malachite green:** Chemicals than can treat and prevent external fungi and parasite infections in farmed fish and in fish eggs. Both have been found to be absorbed into fatty tissues of fish and to have carcinogenic and mutagenic effects in test animals. Some research has even linked them to human cancer. As a result, they are now banned in the United States and Canada, but still used in many other countries.

Farm-raised fish are also given hormones to encourage rapid growth. This allows them to escape their unhealthy environment as quickly as possible—before they get too sick or die. As with growth hormones given to cattle (see chapter 6), they make economic sense. But they may not be so good for us consumers.

Of course, we aren't completely sure about just how big a health risk is posed by certain antibiotics and other drug residues in seafood. But while the science is evolving, we may want to be a little careful.

Keeping Low on POPs and Other Chemicals

ANOTHER RISK ISSUE we need to be aware of when we eat seafood is those persistent toxic chemicals (POPs, already mentioned in connection with fruits and vegetables).

Because toxic chemicals such as PCBs and dioxins are present in *most* of our waterways, fish that live in such contaminated waters build them up in their tissues. In late 2009, the EPA released the final report of the "National Study of Chemical Residues in Lake Fish Tissue," a four-year survey of contaminants in fish from lakes and reservoirs in forty-eight states (excluding Alaska and Hawaii). The results show PCBs and mercury to be present in *all* of the fish samples collected from the five hundred lakes and reservoirs selected for the study. Dioxins and furans were also frequently detected in fish tissues, but were not as prevalent as PCBs.

Let's look at San Francisco Bay as an example. Testing of certain species of sport fish there found five chemical contaminants in addition to mercury to be at "levels of concern"—PCBs, DDT, dieldrin, chlordane, and dioxins. The San Francisco Bay levels are similar to those in Santa Monica Bay. Although the toxic chemical levels in California waterways are frightening, some of these toxic chemicals, such as PCBs, are many times higher in the waterways of other states, as in the Great Lakes region. Such toxic chemicals are also likely to be present in the waterways of countries from which we import our fish, perhaps even in higher concentrations.

Again, you are more at risk from such chemicals if you like to eat larger, older fish, and fish that eat other smaller fish—or if you eat farmed fish such as salmon. Studies have found that farmed salmon tend to have much higher concentrations of toxic substances than do wild salmon. A University of Texas study reported in *Environmental Health Perspectives* in 2010 found salmon to be the most chemically contaminated food product tested, with the highest levels of PCBs among fish. Other studies have also reported high levels of PCBs and dioxins. Is our farmed salmon fit to eat?

A meal or two of heavily chemical-contaminated seafood is unlikely to do us any harm. The danger lies in eating such fish regularly. In that case, the chemicals may build up in our body, some chemicals more than others.

DIOXINS

Take the case of dioxins. Dioxins are a group of chlorinated organic chemicals. They are released unintentionally into the environment through activities such as incineration and fuel combustion. They can also be generated by forest fires and volcanic activity. Dioxins are highly persistent in the environment, including in many of our waterways—and in our fish. Dioxin levels in the environment in North America have been declining as a result of costly cleanup efforts, but they still remain dangerously high in some places. The EPA has gone on record as saying "current exposure levels still remain a concern" and views dioxins as a serious public health threat.

The reason the EPA is concerned is, first, because dioxins are among the most toxic chemicals we know, and second, because we know they bioaccumulate and can stay there for years. In fact, if we were tested, most of us would come up positive for dioxins in our body.

The EPA has classified dioxins as "likely to be human carcinogens." One of the most toxic dioxins—and also one that has been studied most—is TCDD. In 1997, the International Agency for Research on Cancer (IARC) classified several of the TCDDs as a "known human carcinogen." Probably about 10 percent of the dioxins we pick up are TCDDs. Lower levels of dioxin exposure have been linked to a number of health issues, mostly in animal testing. They include birth defects, inability to maintain pregnancy, decreased fertility, spontaneous abortion, birth defects, endometriosis, diabetes, learning disabilities, immune system suppression, lung problems, skin disorders, reduced sperm count, lowered testosterone levels, and more. It is difficult to get reliable results on effects in humans.

Although we can absorb dioxins from several sources, more than 90 percent of human exposure to dioxins is believed to be through the food supply—from the fatty parts of foods such as fish and shellfish, as well from fat in meat and dairy. Fat is bad for our health in more ways than one.

As with mercury, both PCBs and dioxins are a likely to be a special risk to pregnant women, since the unborn child's physical and mental development may be affected, with problems persisting right through school age. In some senses, this risk is worse than the mercury one because PCBs and dioxins can remain stored in the body in a form of half-life for six to ten years, or even longer. So if there is a chance that you may have children in your twenties, start watching your PCBs in your teens.

I also want to briefly mention pink colorants that may be added to trout or salmon feed (as well as to your sausages), but that are also widely present in nature (including in chanterelle mushrooms) and in tanning pills. We may occasionally worry about this issue when we look at that pretty pink farmed salmon in the display counter. Farmed salmon's natural color tends to be grayish white.

We prefer it to be a deep pink, which we associate with wild-caught sockeye salmon. One of the most commonly used dyes to give salmon a pink color is canthaxanthin. This phytochemical has been linked to human retinal damage, although the risk is still poorly understood and more research is needed. The WHO review of the issue and studies that I read do not reach a firm conclusion about risks to humans (or even to the dogs or rats on which the substance was tested). Because of the possibility of health risks, the FDA apparently requires labels on farmed salmon to identify use of coloring. But such labels are hard to find.

Knowing the Natural Toxins

NATURAL TOXINS CAN also occur in seafood. Most originate in tiny organisms in the marine environment. Some can barely affect us, whereas others can be lethal. These toxins will not be destroyed by cooking. One of the trickiest situations occurs if we get a dose of a natural toxin from some tropical fish while overseas. A doctor back home may not diagnose it correctly. Even if he (or she) does, there are few treatments.

The problem with natural toxins in seafood is that we have no warning that they're there. Usually we cannot see, smell, or taste the difference. Fish contaminated with marine toxins can taste delicious. But at least we know that some types of fish and shellfish, certain kinds of waters, and specific times of year are more dangerous than others. Often states such as California post warnings along the seashore during the summer, and many places have quarantine periods for such shellfish as mussels.

Marine toxins tend to be associated with certain fish and shellfish. In the United States, the most common marine toxin–caused illnesses, in order of incidence, are scromboid fish poisoning, ciguatera poisoning, paralytic shellfish poisoning, neurotoxic shellfish poisoning, and amnesic shellfish poisoning. Scromboid fish poisoning is caused differently from the others and is discussed last.

Azaspiracid poisoning, although not as prevalent, is included here because it may be on the increase.

Ciguatera poisoning: The natural neurotoxin ciguatera is most often present in tropical reef fish such as yellowtail, barracuda, grouper, snapper, mackerel, and sea bass, in places such as Hawaii, Virgin Islands, Puerto Rico, and Pacific Islands. In all, some four hundred species of fish have been linked to it, including salmon.

Symptoms occur in a few minutes to thirty hours—usually vomiting, nausea, cramps, headache, muscle aches, sweating, and diarrhea. Symptoms can also include itching, dizziness, weakness, a "pins and needles" sensation, hot-cold reversal in the mouth, hallucinations, and an unusual taste. It is rarely fatal. Ciguatera poisoning can produce neuro-psychiatric problems for weeks and sometimes for years afterward, including fatigue and depression. They could be mistaken for chronic fatigue syndrome. It has been suggested that there may be a connection between the two.

Paralytic shellfish poisoning (PSP): PSP toxins may be present in the dark digestive organs of most shellfish (oysters, mussels, clams, cockles, crabs, and scallops) in cooler waters, including in New England and California. The FDA occasionally warns consumers not to eat the tomalley of Maine lobsters (the soft green substance inside the lobster's head) for this reason, as it did in July 2008. The lobster meat itself remains safe to eat. PSP is not destroyed by cooking.

PSP symptoms can occur fifteen minutes to ten hours after eating, and start with numbness or tingling in the face, followed by dizziness, nausea, headache and loss of muscular coordination. One may also experience a floating sensation. In the worst cases, paralysis and respiratory failure can occur. It can be fatal.

Neurotoxic shellfish poisoning: Can be caused by mussels, oysters, and clams from the Gulf of Mexico and the Atlantic coast of the Southern states.

Symptoms occur quickly, usually one to three hours after eating, and include gastrointestinal symptoms, tingling and numbness in the mouth, arms and legs, and loss of coordination. Temperature reversal can also occur, as with ciguatera poisoning. It is rarely fatal.

Amnesic shellfish poisoning: This poisoning occurs when **demoic acid** accumulates in the digestive organs and meat of mussels, oysters, and razor clams, and in the viscera of sardines, anchovies, crab, and lobster. One of the best-known incidents occurred in Canada in 1987 as a result of consumption of contaminated blue mussels (resulting in over two hundred illnesses and at least four deaths). Specific control measures have been implemented since then.

Symptoms such as gastrointestinal distress can occur within twenty-four hours and be followed by others such as headache, dizziness, and disorientation. Permanent short-term memory loss can result. In severe poisoning, there may also be seizures, focal weakness or paralysis, and death. Demoic acid is not as heat stable as PSP, but is not completely inactivated by cooking, either.

Azaspiracid shellfish poisoning: Can originate in shellfish, such as mussels. The toxin was only identified in 1995. A recent recall by the FDA involved frozen cooked mussels imported from Ireland. Mussels from Ireland have also caused outbreaks in other countries.

Symptoms include gastrointestinal distress but can also include neurological problems, including paralysis and even death in extreme cases.

Scromboid poisoning: Also known as histamine fish poisoning, this is different from the above toxins. It occurs when certain fish spoil as a result of incorrect handling and storage. The resulting histamine proteins can cause serious allergic reactions in people who eat the fish. Scromboid poisoning has mainly been associated with such fish as tuna, mahimahi, bluefish, and mackerel. Usually few people are involved in any poisoning incidents. In one outbreak in Pennsylvania, four people became ill with it after eating tuna-spinach salad at the same restaurant. In New Mexico, a husband and wife became ill with scromboid poisoning after grilling previously frozen mahimahi that had been imported from Taiwan. These are just two examples.

A reaction can occur between two minutes and a few hours. Symptoms include flushing of the face, a rash like sunburn, a bad metallic taste or burning in the mouth, sweating, headache, diarrhea, abdominal pain, and vomiting. The symptoms can be more severe in people who are taking certain kinds of medicines that slow down breakdown of histamine by the liver.

Even though there is no way you can always tell when seafood is contaminated with a natural toxin, there are certain rules you can follow. For instance, do not eat barracuda, especially if it comes from the Caribbean. If you want to be extra careful, you may also want to avoid other fish if it comes from tropical waters, such as grouper, snapper, mackerel, mullet, and sea bass, because they are more likely to be risky. Before collecting shellfish, check advisories (search your local health department online and also check advisories posted at the shore) for alerts about "red tide" or other algae conditions. Should you believe you have ingested such natural toxins, induced vomiting could help—that is, if you catch it soon enough. In some cases, illness occurs anyway. As always, be careful of dehydration.

Read Those Labels

Country of Origin Labeling (COOL)

As noted earlier, retailers and their suppliers in the United States and Canada now have to label the origins of their fish and shellfish. In practice, this requirement becomes more complicated with seafood than with foods such as produce. For instance, in the case of farm-raised seafood, if the country of origin is stated as the United States, then it must be derived only from fish or shellfish hatched, raised, harvested, and processed in the United States. COOL requires that it must "not have undergone substantial transformation outside the U.S." In the case of wild fish or shellfish, if the United States is used as the "country of origin," then the seafood must be exclusively harvested in U.S. waters or by a U.S.-flagged vessel and processed in the United States or aboard a U.S.-flagged vessel. Again, any transformation has to have taken place in the United States. In sum, for seafood to be labeled as originating in the United States, it has to be American all the way.

Organic

Presently, there are no "organic" standards in place for seafood in the United States or Canada. But it is on some labels, right? Quite often *imported* seafood is labeled "organic." Store notices on fresh fish (a label stuck into fresh fish or on the tray) sometimes also say that the product is "organic" or "organically fed." At least in some cases, such labels are placed on fish that are given hormones and antibiotics, although they may be primarily organically fed—that is, given a lower proportion of fish in their feed. They may also live in less crowded conditions, although this cannot be guaranteed. At time of writing, organic regulations for fish and shellfish are in the works. In the meantime, take any "organic" labeling on seafood with a grain of salt. In case it makes you feel better, official complaints have been filed with the USDA to prevent the use of this label on imported seafood.

Use-by Date

Most canned food, including canned fish, now has a "best if used-by date." So do packaged smoked salmon and other such seafood products. A can of tuna can have a "best-by" date as much as four years away from when you buy it. In case you have wondered about that other mysterious number on the can—this is when it was packaged. Canned food manufacturers have different coding systems. Canned seafood should be stored at temperatures no higher than about 75°F and eaten no later than the "best-by" or "use-by" date.

But What About . . . ?

How can I tell if the fish I am buying is fresh?

In the case of fish, make sure the whole fish or fillet is shiny and looks firm. Look at the way the seafood is presented: It should be refrigerated or on ice, and fresh seafood should not be next to cooked seafood. Whole fish should have clear, bulging eyes (except in the case of walleye and a few other fish, which have cloudy eyes) and the gills should be bright pink or red. You may even want to ask your fish vendor to press the fish flesh, to make sure it springs back. (If it is on an open display counter, do it yourself when no one is looking.) The fish should also smell fresh, not too "fishy"—and not like your bathroom cleaner. (Household cleaners frequently contain ammonia, which smell can also be associated with rotting fish.) Fish fillets should be moist (not dry or brownish at the edges). In the case of frozen seafood, make sure it does not have freezer burn and that the frozen fish has a thick glaze of ice on it.

If children eat a lot of fish, are they getting too much mercury?

There are slight differences of opinion, but I would say that you need not worry about mercury if your children are eating the fish in form of fish sticks, fast-food fish sandwiches, wild salmon, sardines, rainbow trout, crawfish, fresh tilapia, or such other low-mercury fish (see page 107). For tuna sandwiches, use only "light" tuna. Varying the seafood children eat will help to protect them from a buildup of other dangerous substances as well. Also, do not give them huge portions of the fish. Some experts suggest no more than three ounces of fish for younger children and four to five ounces for older children (the weight of the raw fish). For more information, go to www.kidsafeseafood.org.

Is it a problem to eat a lot of high-mercury fish during a week's vacation at the beach?

No. Not unless you are pregnant. Just keep very low on mercury for the next few weeks, and it will gradually be eliminated from your body.

Am I safer from bacteria and parasites if I make sushi at home than if I eat it out?

Sorry—it could be the opposite. You will only be safer with homemade sushi if you are very careful. Make sure you buy only "sushi-grade" or "sashimi-grade" fish. These labels can only be used for fish that has been commercially frozen according to FDA regulations. It is not the sort of thing that can be done in your home freezer.

Smart Ways to Reduce Your Risks

SEAFOOD IS ONE of our riskiest foods, particularly for pregnant women and children. This has a lot to do with our eating more farmed seafood, and especially farmed fish and shellfish imported from countries with very polluted waters and poorly enforced regulations. Some of our favorite fish and shellfish, such as shrimp, tuna, and salmon, could be among the riskiest. The general rule for protecting yourself and your family when eating seafood is: "Know your fish or shellfish, cook it well, and watch how much you eat." But you could also keep seven simple rules in mind (see sidebar).

SEVEN SIMPLE SAFETY RULES FOR SEAFOOD

Let's sum it all up. When choosing or eating seafood, remember the generally applicable seven simple rules (although with exceptions):

1. Raw is risky.
2. Wild is usually safer than farmed.
3. Small is usually safer than large.
4. Domestic is usually safer than imported.
5. Fish fat and fatty fish are best avoided.
6. Dark parts of shellfish are more dangerous than light parts.
7. Diversification is a good idea.

But all this does not mean you should give up eating fish. People all over the world have been eating fish for a long time, and the majority have not suffered any ill effects (or, of course, there is no evidence that it was the fish that did it). Besides, there are smart decisions you can make that will lower your risk. If there is any food about which being an educated consumer pays off, seafood is it.

Be careful when fishing or collecting your own shellfish. Always read the fish advisories before going out, including those for lakes and streams. If the fish you catch smells of ammonia, throw it out, but warning smells are not always present if fish carry natural toxins. Make sure not to collect potentially toxic shellfish during quarantine periods (mussels are a key one to watch out for, because they develop toxicity more quickly). Don't collect mollusks immediately after a storm, and avoid doing it near sewage or other outlets or culverts running down to the beach, or near grazing animals or boats that may discharge sewage. If a friend shares a catch, tactfully ask where it was caught and check the advisory before eating. When catching your own fish, gut and clean them as soon as the fish are dead, so that any parasites in the gut don't migrate into the flesh. Immediately place the fish on ice in a cooler to keep them fresh.

Buy the freshest fish and shellfish. If you buy only one kind of food from the most reputable dealers, make it seafood—and even then, check to make sure it is fresh (see page 122 for how to check). If a particular fish is on sale, be doubly careful. (That was my mistake last week: I threw out the fish when I came home.) Get the fish into your refrigerator as quickly as possible (buy it last). If you live more than one hundred miles from the coast, you may want to think twice before buying fresh fish. Frozen fish is often safest these days, as it is quickly flash-frozen on the boat, although it won't usually taste as good as fresh fish. In fact, much of our so-called fresh fish is actually previously frozen. Fresh mollusks in the shell such as clams, mussels, oysters, or scallops should always be alive when you buy them. The shells should either be tightly closed or should close when you tap them or put them on ice. Throw away any that do not close.

Buy wild or domestic farm-raised fish when you can. Find out where your fish comes from, and buy domestic if you can. The evidence suggests that imported farmed fish may be more unsafe in terms of the chemicals, drugs, metals, or such other unhealthy substances. But even in the case of American farmed fish, you may want to buy "organically fed" when you can, to avoid drug residues. Ask your fish vendor three specific questions: (1) Where are these fish from? (2) Have they been organically fed? and (3) Are they free of antibiotics and hormones? Of course, the vendor may not always know; in which case; ask the manager or store owner—or, change vendors. Of course, as long as they are species considered low mercury—and affordable—buy wild fish, but even then choose the nonpredators or smaller ones of a species.

Store seafood correctly. Keep fresh seafood in the coldest part of the refrigerator (such as the meat drawer), in the wrapper in which you bought it and with a layer of ice if you plan to keep it more than a few hours. Smoked fish and marinated herrings or similar fish should also be refrigerated to slow down the multiplication of bacteria. Canned fish does not have to be refrigerated until opened. Do not put cooked seafood back in a container that has held raw seafood. Also, do not refreeze a previously frozen fish (remember—many "fresh" fish are previously frozen, so they shouldn't be refrozen, either). You should not store fish or shellfish in the refrigerator for more than two days without cooking, even if on ice. If you suddenly find some fish in the refrigerator that you forgot about, throw it out and eat beans, rather than risk becoming ill. Don't even give it to your cat.

Prepare seafood safely. If seafood has been stored in the refrigerator, remove it only when you are ready to cook it. When thawing frozen fish or shellfish, thaw it in the refrigerator (be patient—it may take as long as a day). To speed things up, you may want to use the defrost setting on your oven, if you have one. Or defrost the fish or shellfish in a sealed plastic bag in a bowl of water, changing the water and keeping an eye on it. The fact to remember is that you need to keep seafood out of the "temperature danger zone" between 40° and 140°F within which bacteria multiply most rapidly.

Cook fish thoroughly. Cook seafood as soon as possible. When cooking fish, allow about ten minutes for each inch of thickness, turning over halfway. If cooking in foil or sauce, add at least five minutes. Before serving, always check the thickest part of the fish to make sure that the flesh is opaque, not translucent. When cooking fillets, cook to an internal temperature of at least 145°F. (This is where a meat thermometer comes in handy.) If you are the lucky owner of a home smoker for fish, remember that light smoking will probably not kill all microbes, including parasites. Nor is marinating fish or shellfish in lemon juice or vinegar a guaranteed "kill" step. Steam, broil, bake, or grill your larger fish rather than frying them, as that will get rid of more of the fat where many toxins accumulate.

Cook mollusks thoroughly. Wash them first. When boiling, make sure all mollusks are being heated evenly. Watch for the shells opening, and then cook for an additional three to five minutes. If steaming, cook for four to nine minutes. But don't overcook, or the mollusks will lose their flavor. The same applies to shellfish such as shrimp (cooking times, three to eight minutes, depending on size). After cooking mollusks, check all of them and discard any that have not opened. If you are discarding more than one in ten, don't buy from that store anymore.

Eat selectively. Avoid eating the larger, predatory fish as much as possible, to reduce your exposure to mercury, other toxic chemicals, and parasites. Do not eat the fatty part of fish, or eat very fatty fish such as carp and catfish, as this is where many toxic chemicals such as dioxins and PCBs tend to be concentrated. (Remember, this does not help remove any mercury.) When eating fish such as salmon, particularly farmed salmon (which are more fatty than wild salmon), remove the fatty skin and darker meat, which could help you reduce any PCBs by about 50 percent. In fact, some scientists who have studied toxic chemicals in it recommend that you limit your consumption of farmed salmon to one, or at most two, meals a month. To reduce your exposure to toxins when eating shellfish, remove all dark parts from mussels, oysters, and clams before eating them, and do not eat the organs or viscera of lobster or crab, as this is where toxic substances are likely to be highest. Remember, cooking will not destroy natural toxins or histamine in fish. Avoid regularly eating any dish that is made from whole fish, such as bouillabaisse. Such dishes usually contain parts of fish where chemicals tend to concentrate.

Reduce your risks if you eat raw or lightly cooked seafood. If you absolutely insist on eating raw fish (and I have to admit that I love ceviche), make sure the fish used has been commercially frozen first. Don't be afraid to ask, if you are either buying the fish or eating out. But even then, remember that there is an element of risk. If you really insist on eating raw oysters, you may want to make sure that they have been irradiated, that is, if you don't mind irradiation. My research suggests that some suppliers of oysters are also much safer than others.

Eat restaurant seafood carefully. Only eat fish, especially shellfish or any raw fish dish, at highly reliable restaurants. Always ask where the seafood comes from, if farmed or wild, and whether it has been frozen. (If you are told that the raw fish to be used for your ceviche or sashimi has *not* been frozen, run.) Make sure the cooked seafood is properly cooked (watch out especially for any translucent salmon). If not, send it back. In the case of mollusks, as always, discard any on your plate that have unopened shells. Complain and ask for your money back if there are too many that haven't opened!

Be super careful if you are pregnant or giving seafood to your young children. You would be smart to avoid raw fish dishes such as sushi or sashimi, or eating raw mollusks, especially raw oysters. You should also avoid high-mercury fish, premade/store- or restaurant-made seafood salads or sandwiches, and ready-to-eat seafood such as smoked fish, mussels, and oysters (unless canned). If you are thinking of becoming pregnant and love fish, try phasing out tuna and other high-mercury fish, replacing them with lower-mercury varieties such as salmon, tilapia, shrimp, catfish, and others, to lower the accumulated mercury levels in your body. Remember, that to completely eliminate toxic chemicals such as dioxins and PCBs, your body could need six to ten years, or even longer. That requires considerable long-term planning. Pregnant women are probably smart to avoid all shellfish for those nine months. For children, see the answer in the previous section to the question about mercury, and remember to not give them the fatty part of any fish.

6

Meat and Poultry

ONE OF MY most vivid childhood memories is of watching chickens being slaughtered. Nowadays very few chickens or other food animals meet their end on small farms, with a seven-year-old child watching as the ax comes down. Factory farming has changed almost everything about meat production. But has it made meat safer? We continue to have regular alerts and large recalls. Often the cause is bacteria such as *E. coli* or *Salmonella*. Factory farming has also brought us longer-term worries about hormones and antibiotics in our hamburger or steak. Their use may keep the meat prices down—and help the industry profits—but are they worth it? On top of all this, in recent years we have come frighteningly close to global scares such as mad cow disease. And that's just the short list of what could be in our dinner.

In some ways, our meat and poultry are safer than they used to be. Over the years, theirs has become one of the most heavily regulated food industries. In other ways, it is probably worse. If you look at meat and poultry in terms of the number of cases of food poisoning, these **animal products** are safer to eat than are fresh fruit, vegetables, and fish—unless, of course, we eat them raw or undercooked (as in the case of underdone hamburgers or steak tartare). But cooking only takes care of some of the more obvious problems, not all—mainly the short-term food poisoning risks. In fact, one could argue that long-term consumption of meat and poultry may now expose us to more health hazards than before—and not only in terms of nutritional risks. In addition, there is the fact that our food animals could be responsible, either directly or indirectly, for some of the hazards in our other foods—including our salad and our fish.

What We Eat

Most Americans, except for vegetarians and vegans, eat a lot of meat—an average of over two hundred pounds a year. Canadians have been found to eat significantly less, but still far above the global average. In both the United States and Canada, meat consumption has increased over the years. But meat preferences have changed. There has been a general shift toward eating less red meat and more poultry (and fish). In fact, chicken is now the most popular animal product in the American diet, followed by beef, and then pork. As for how we eat it—no surprise—much of the meat and poultry eaten in North America is in the form of fast food. We are also eating more in the form of quick and convenient meats, such as deli meats and hot dogs.

Let's take a closer look at meat and poultry consumption patterns in the United States.

Poultry. Americans are now eating about twice as much chicken as in 1970—close to ninety pounds of chicken per year. Chicken's neutral taste, easy preparation, and low cost contribute to its success. Turkey is the next most popular poultry. Other domestic poultry (such as duck and goose), and more exotic poultry (such as guinea hen, partridge, peafowl, pigeons, grouse, pheasants, ostrich, emu, and quail) are far behind. Overall, as long as it is cooked well, poultry is relatively safe to eat. In fact, it may be more dangerous to *prepare* your raw chicken than to eat chicken (more about that later).

Beef. Americans average about sixty-seven pounds of beef per person each year. The most popular form of beef eaten in America is ground meat. It is also the riskiest. Ground meat is used to make our favorite food—the hamburger—and for such other foods as taco fillings, pasta sauce, and meatballs. Steaks are next in popularity. Even when eating out, we tend to order ground beef meals more than half the time. Lower price is a factor, as well as taste.

Pork. Pork is the most widely eaten meat in the world, but in America it ranks only third. In addition to consuming pork chops and roasts, we frequently eat small quantities of pork in such foods as pizza toppings, lunch meats, hot dogs, ham, and bacon. The average per person consumption is about fifty pounds of pork a year. Thanks to a clever marketing campaign by the National Pork Board, we tend to think of it as "the other white meat" although, strictly speaking, it is red meat . . . or, if you like, "pink"—in between beef and chicken, in terms of myoglobin (the protein that defines red meat). These days, pork is a lot leaner than it used to be.

Lamb, mutton, goat, and more exotic meats. Although more unusual meats may be standard fare among some ethnic groups in our vast melting pot, the average American eats only about one pound of lamb or mutton per year, down from about five pounds in the 1960s. (Compare this to the average New Zealander's fifty or so pounds a year and the Australian's thirty-seven pounds.) We eat even less goat, although it has been gaining in popularity. Only a small percentage of Americans ever eat game, such as rabbit or venison, or more exotic meats, such as ostrich, elk, moose, wild boar, buffalo, bison, kangaroo, camel, guinea pigs, and even alligator, snake, and gecko. You would be surprised by what is available if you want it, at gourmet markets, online, and on a few select restaurant menus.

Who Keeps It Safe?

MEAT SAFETY REGULATION has been a focus of concern again and again over the years, up to and including the present time. The slaughterhouse—the riskiest point—has received special attention from the beginning. More recently, the riskiness of ready-to-eat meats has received increased recognition, especially in Canada. We now find a greater emphasis on the prevention of problems, which is a good thing.

In Canada, HC—as usual—is responsible for establishing policies and safety standards, while CFIA is responsible for actually making sure that both domestic and imported meats are safe and wholesome. Its responsibilities include inspection of the slaughter and processing facilities for meat products, in collaboration with provincial authorities.

Let's take a closer look at some of the aspects of regulation in the United States, where the USDA/FSIS is responsible for ensuring that meat and poultry products are "safe, wholesome, and accurately labeled." The agency must inspect each animal we eat when it is alive and as a carcass, to make sure it is disease free. The Animal and Plant Health Inspection Service (APHIS) monitors animal health. Again, state-level agencies cooperate and do much of the usual hands-on work of inspections, educating the public, overseeing recalls, and so forth.

These organizations do what they can with their available resources. Among other things, these government regulators decide whether and how hormones and antibiotics can be used for our food animals; which bacteria, in what numbers, can be present in fresh meat or poultry; and what levels of toxic substances in our meat will not harm us.

The red tape of just which U.S. government agency does what would be almost comical, were our health not in the balance. For example, the USDA/FSIS is not only responsible for the safety of fresh meats but also for any processed products such as frozen foods, stews, and such items as meat or chicken pizzas, if they contain *sufficient amounts* of meat or poultry. "Sufficient" amounts? Yes, it seems that a pizza that has a raw meat or poultry content of greater than 3 percent, or a cooked meat or poultry content greater than 2 percent, would be inspected by USDA/FSIS. If it has less, the FDA is responsible. Also, the FSIS only oversees the "traditional" meats. Exotic and game meats are instead overseen by the FDA (I have no idea why).

The industry's response to new safety measures has not always been positive. Unfortunately, increased regulation of any kind, including safety regulation, tends to be most costly for the small producers and processors. New safety measures can even drive them out of business. Often, big industry does not mind additional safety measures quite as much, particularly if they are likely to avoid costly outbreaks—and concentrate more business in their hands.

TRY REGULATING A SAUSAGE

If you think that ensuring our steaks are safe to eat is difficult, think of the sausage. The sausage is a very complex product that results from numerous tricky steps. About two hundred types of sausage are sold in the United States alone—fresh, fresh cooked, smoked, dry and semidry, hard and soft sausages. Some sausages are uncooked, some partly cooked, others completely cooked and ready-to-eat.

Sausage manufacturers have their secret formulas for making sausages, and the process can vary considerably. The basic steps include chopping or grinding the meat(s) and mixing it with other ingredients such as spices; stuffing the mixture into a tubelike container or casing; and processing by cooking, smoking, fermenting, curing or air-drying the sausage. "Good" mold and "good" bacteria play a part in the making of certain kinds of sausages.

The USDA/FSIS has regulations that prescribe what a sausage may or may not contain, and checks to make sure that these regulations are followed (as much as resources allow). These regulations specify what kind of meat or poultry can be put into the sausage (most sausages use meat scraped off the animal's skeleton), the amount and type of other ingredients in it (such as soy protein, whey, or milk powder), the amount of fat in the sausage (it can be no more than 30 percent), and the type of casing used (natural—such as the intestine of an animal—or artificial). When inspectors visit a sausage plant, they check to see whether the plant is following safe procedures, assess whether plant conditions are sanitary, inspect the sausage ingredients, check records, and take test samples of sausages. But their visits are often too short, the tests are not always performed, and the inspections never cover all possible hazards.

Are you surprised that sausages are a commonly contaminated food product? Anything in them could be the culprit ingredient—one of the meats used, other components such as milk powder, and even the spices. Or the source of contamination could be one of those plant workers or pieces of equipment. Inspecting a sausage is far from easy.

Again as with other foods, the resource-poor government is trying to get the meat industry to take over more of the responsibility for safety. The earlier-mentioned HACCP is playing a role in this. And again, as usual, although the government tries to make sure that the meat and meat products that enter the country are unadulterated and uncontaminated, properly packaged, undamaged, and accurately labeled, only a small percentage of imported meat or meat products can actually be inspected, and an even smaller percentage actually tested. But take comfort in knowing that for a country to be allowed to send meat or poultry into the United States, it has to prove that it can meet the U.S. standards. Using both documents and on-site review, the USDA/FSIS evaluates the exporting country's laws, regulations, and infrastructure in terms of sanitation, animal disease, slaughter and processing, residues, and enforcement. The FSIS also inspects foreign meat-processing plants—when it can—to make sure that everything continues to be fine. If not, it can suspend imports from the country or a particular plant or suspend a specific product.

But in actual practice, resources are always a constraint on what government can do, and enforcement power everywhere is a problem—in the case of both domestic and imported meats.

Kill Those Bacteria

BACTERIA CAN EASILY get into meat, right from the start. Try slaughtering an animal or bird in a sanitary way, and you will realize how difficult it is. Animals carry bacteria in their intestines. Bacteria also build up on their hides and hooves during transport and as they nervously wait for their turn to come up at the slaughterhouse. Washing will not remove all of the germs—any more than it does with your apple. The trick during slaughter is to prevent bacteria that are present on the skin and inside the animal from landing on the raw meat that is then sent to your store.

Many bacteria in food animals can be dangerous to humans, but the cow, chicken, or pig may not show signs of illness. Even if inspectors—who are supposed to be present at slaughterhouses at all times—do both their live animal and carcass inspections properly, some bacteria will still get through. You can't see bacteria. Testing does not pick up all of them, either. Just a few can be enough to cause problems, and these pesky microorganisms hold the world's record for reproduction. Under the right conditions—a nice nutritious environment, as in meat, and temperatures between 40° and 140°F—some of them double in number every twenty minutes. This means that a single bacteria can multiply to over a million bacteria in less than seven hours.

The number and regularity of bacteria-contaminated meat incidents prove that raw meat remains risky. The one we hear most about is *E. coli* O157:H7 (see sidebar). No doubt about it, this bacterium and its other Shiga-like toxin–producing relatives (such as *E. coli* O145), are about the worst.

ENJOY YOUR HAMBURGER WITH A TOUCH OF *E. COLI*

E. coli O157:H7 is one of the most deadly microbes you can come across in your food, and is one of the most deadly strains of *E. coli* bacteria (many of the others are perfectly harmless to adults). The U.S. government estimates that *E. coli* O157:H7 causes about 700,000 American illnesses a year. It turns up frequently in our meat. Even when it is in other kinds of food—such as dairy, leafy greens, spinach, or raw sprouts (see pages 184, 49, and 240)—cross-contamination with meat or meat animals is often the cause. Of course, you can also get this form of *E. coli* just from hugging a cow or from your swimming pool. It is everywhere.

For those of us who are reasonably healthy, a dose of this bacterium just means two to ten days of misery and perhaps even some hemorrhagic diarrhea. It is possible to have virtually no symptoms at all—but to pass on the bacterium to your best friend, your boss, or your child. In vulnerable people, and particularly young children, life-threatening hemolytic uremic syndrome (HUS) can develop. Such complications happen in about one case out of fifteen.

A very common way to catch *E. coli* O157:H7 is through eating undercooked hamburgers. The rarer they are, the more you are at risk. The food will look, taste, and smell as it always does—delicious. The kind of burger meat you buy and where you buy it from are also important factors. Bacteria risks in hamburger meat are due to the low-quality meats, the mixing with other ingredients (such as beef fat), and the processing steps (such as grinding) involved. Both frozen and fresh meat can carry *E. coli*. You don't even have to eat the meat to catch this germ. The very act of preparing a hamburger can be dangerous in itself.

Yes, government and industry have made major efforts in recent years to eliminate *E. coli* O157:H7 completely from our food. Currently, the American government is starting a special initiative to reduce risks of *E. coli* O157:H7's turning up in beef, and particularly in hamburger meat. There is zero tolerance for the bacterium; this is one contaminant that doesn't have an "acceptable" number. But clearly *E. coli* O157:H7 has not got the message. It is still turning up in our beef, as well as in other ground meats and poultry. In just a twelve-month period, June 2009 to May 2010, eight recalls were recorded for *E. coli* O157:H7 meat or meat products. There were twice as many involving ground beef as for any other kind of meat.

Any uninvited appearance of *E. coli* O157:H7 becomes a crisis for the company involved, as well as for the victims. In some cases, the firm does not survive, as happened in the case of the safety-conscious seventy-year-old family-owned Topps Meat Company after it had to recall twenty-two million pounds of its frozen hamburger patties.

The source of the famous *E. coli* O157:H7 contamination of Jack in the Box hamburgers, back in the 1990s, was never conclusively identified. It might have entered in the slaughterhouse or in the kitchen. The meat industry blamed the food chain for not cooking its hamburgers enough. The food chain blamed the industry for providing it with bad meat. So it goes.

Toxin-producing species *E. coli* are, of course, not the only bacteria that can turn up in our meat or poultry. There are also plenty of others, including *Campylobacter jejuni* (in beef and poultry); *Clostridium perfringens* (in beef, chicken, turkey, and pork); *E. coli* O157:H7 (in ground beef, ground chicken, and pork); *Listeria monocytogenes* (in ready-to-eat meat products); *Salmonella* spp. (in beef, pork, and poultry); *Staphylococcus aureus* (in beef, pork, and poultry); and *Yersinia enterocolitica* (in pork). Of the twenty-two U.S. meat recalls in 2009 that were linked to bacteria—one every month except for March—eleven were caused by *E. coli* O157:H7, seven by *Listeria* bacteria, and four were linked to *Salmonella*.

Studies have found that, in fact, *the large majority* of raw meat and poultry carries at least some disease-causing bacteria. Take chicken—our favorite. The most common bacterial contaminants of raw and RTE chicken are *Salmonella enteritidis*, *Campylobacter jejuni*, *Staphylococcus aureus*, and *Listeria monocytogenes*. A report released by *Consumer Reports* in late 2006 found that fully 83 percent of the chickens it tested in stores in twenty-three states carried *Campylobacter, Salmonella,* or both. (Naturally the National Chicken Council said that the *Consumer Reports* figures were "greatly exaggerated.") The CDC estimates that each year as many as 1.1 million Americans are sickened by undercooked chicken that harbor bacteria or by other food that raw chicken or its juices have touched—usually salads or other vegetables that are eaten raw. The U.S. government has gotten the message. In May 2010, it announced new, stricter performance standards for poultry establishments, in hopes these will reduce the *Salmonella* and *Campylobacter* in young chickens and turkeys and eliminate tens of thousands of illnesses a year.

Then there is the issue of bacterial contamination of deli meats, other RTE products such as cooked pizzas and meat spreads, and ready-to-cook meat and poultry products such as breaded chicken breasts. In their case, the bacteria usually enter during processing—not at slaughter. Contaminated processing equipment or facilities can be the cause, as can be bacteria-carrying plant workers. The culprit bacterium in such foods is usually *Listeria*. Remember—*Listeria* bacteria are very dangerous in late stages of pregnancy (see chapter 7 for more information on this, especially the sidebar on page 186) and for other people with a weakened immune system. The high-end estimate is that 30 percent of meat plant workers carry this bacterium. Also, *Listeria* can survive and even multiply in the refrigerator, where deli meats are supposedly safely stored.

The presence of *Listeria* bacteria in ready-to-eat meats (and other foods) is difficult to prevent. Both the U.S. and Canadian governments have taken measures to control it over recent years, particularly at meat processing plants. Obviously, these efforts have not had much effect—at least, not yet, as outbreaks continue. In 2010 there were several large recalls both in Canada and the United States involving *Listeria* in RTE deli meats and sausages. In two cases, contaminated meat products had been exported by companies based in Canada to the United States.

Cooking is of course the essential step in avoiding any bacteria in meat, because the large majority are killed at high temperatures (see page 173). Actually, Americans *are* reported to cook/order hamburgers and steaks to be more fully cooked than they used to do both at home and in restaurants. But people with high food-risk ratings may even want to cook their RTE luncheon meats. Much as we may enjoy them, barbecues, which sometimes result in unevenly cooked meat, are also best avoided by people at risk, such as pregnant women (by all means, attend these events, but take along your own sandwich).

The Superbug Issue

WE ALL FEAR "superbugs"—or bacteria that are highly resistant to antibiotics. They are growing in number and constitute a major threat to world health. Overprescription of antibiotics by the medical profession is partly responsible. So are our modern food-animal production practices.

Superbugs are much more deadly than "normal" bacteria. The CDC estimates that about half of deaths from infectious diseases are caused by such antibiotic-resistant bacteria. There are others besides the highly publicized MRSA. Many people wrongly believe that such superbugs are only involved in hospital-acquired infections. That is not so. You can also acquire them in other ways—from just a small cut on your hand while you play tennis or football, or from your food.

How are animal production practices encouraging antibiotic-resistant bacteria? The profit-focus of industrialized livestock production has a lot to do with it. Crowded, unsanitary conditions increase the chances of large outbreaks of disease (as they also do in the case of farmed fish; see page 111). One chicken comes down with a case of infectious *E. coli*, and soon the whole flock has it. It is the same as with children in schools and adults in institutional settings such as nursing homes. This is where subtherapeutic (preventive) use of antibiotics comes in. Regular, small doses of certain antibiotics given in feed of broiler chickens, cattle, pigs and so on, helps to keep them well and growing better. Such use of antibiotics has been standard practice in the United States and Canada for years.

No matter what the benefits of this practice, it has a very serious downside. Such low-level, regular use of antibiotics helps to develop bacterial resistance (more so than brief therapeutic use does). The tougher bacteria inside the bird or animal's intestine learn to live with the antibiotics, multiply, and basically take over, while the weaker bacteria succumb. Increasingly, resistant members of the *E. coli, Salmonella, Staphylococcus,* and *Campylobacter* species are found in our meat and poultry products. Many have resistance to those antibiotics we rely on to cure any infections we have. They can be happily alive inside the animal or bird as it goes to slaughter. It would not matter quite so much if these bacteria were just developing resistance to veterinary drugs that are not related to the antibiotics that we humans rely on. But unfortunately, some "medically important" antibiotics *are* being used in producing that chicken or cow that we eat.

If it is dangerous, why is the practice still ongoing in North America? Europe recognized the risks back in 2001 and banned the subtherapeutic use of any antibiotics that were important in human medicine. In some progressive European countries, such as Denmark, farmers had voluntarily taken action against it even earlier. Action against the practice in the United States has been slower. But such continuing use of antibiotics *has* been questioned by a number of prestigious organizations, such as the American Public Health Association (APHA), the American Medical Association (AMA), and the American Society for Microbiology (ASM). The CDC has urged caution. Even major companies, including Perdue, Tyson Foods, and Foster Farms, and fast-food chains such as McDonald's and Wendy's, have taken the issue seriously.

It may end up being a step-by-step battle, where one medically significant antibiotic is withdrawn from use at a time. But in each such case, it could take years. Removing the drug Baytril from being used to prevent illness and promote growth in chickens and turkey was the first such victory in the United States. Baytril is from the same fluoroquinolone class of antibiotics as Cipro (ciproflaxin), which is the drug of choice for treatment of a number of bacterial infections in humans, including around a million U.S. illnesses caused each year by *Campylobacter* bacteria (which may be present in about half of chickens). Even after the government agreed that Baytril was helping to develop human resistance of *Campylobacter* to Cipro, it took a five-year legal battle (2000–2005) to ban its use, while Bayer Corporation protested the decision. The pharmaceutical and meat industries are powerful and have deep pockets to fight any measure they don't like. More recently, the FDA has indicated that it may take a general move toward prohibiting unnecessary use of medically significant antibiotics in animal production. Let's hope it doesn't back down under industry pressure.

Such antibiotic use not only contributes to industry profits but also helps to keep our meat prices down (the same argument is given for hormone use—see page 143). Supporters of the practice say that it is both necessary and safe. I disagree. As someone who literally watched antibiotic resistance developing among bacteria several decades ago and expressed concern then against antibiotic overuse, I feel this is one of the most important public health issues we face today. If I needed reminding, I just need to think of those people I currently know who are battling infections of such antibiotic-resistant bacteria—and have been doing so for years: one close relative and two friends; three people at the moment. In five years' time I may know five, or even ten. The number of victims of superbugs is increasing every day.

If anything should drive you to avoiding contaminants in your meat and poultry, the fear of superbugs should. None of us wants to be the next victim.

. . .

Good-bye Pesky Parasites

As IN THE case of seafood, parasites can also hide in meat and poultry products. From there they can pass to those who consume them. Pork can carry parasites such as *Trichinella spiralis*, which causes trichinosis, and *Taenia solium*, or "pork hookworm." Beef can be contaminated with *Taenia saginata*, or "beef tapeworm." The parasite *Haemonchus contortus* (called "barberpole worm" because it has red and white swirls like old-fashioned barber poles) is a common problem for sheep and goat producers. The tiny parasite *Toxoplasma gondii* (see page 58) can also turn up in beef, pork, and even poultry.

But nowadays parasites in North American meat and poultry are a much lower risk than they used to be, thanks to safety measures being taken by the industry. In fact, we may be as much at risk from getting a dose of an antiparasitic drug from our steak as we are for catching a tapeworm. But because some parasites in our food animals are developing resistance to livestock deworming drugs, these critters could become a bigger problem in the future. And, of course, in some regions outside the United States, these parasites are still a problem. We may find ourselves bringing them back from our tropical vacation, together with our suntan.

Should Growth Hormones Worry Us?

GROWTH HORMONES (HORMONAL growth promoters—HGPs) are a very controversial issue everywhere, including in North America. In the United States, they are widely used in beef cattle and lamb production, but not allowed to be used for poultry, pork, veal, or exotic meat production. At least two thirds of beef on the U.S. market—maybe more—are reported to come from cattle that have been given HGPs. Beef producers give their animals HGPs to encourage rapid growth with less feed and to make meat leaner.

Obviously, this boosts their profits. As with subtherapeutic use of antibiotics, one could also argue that it also gives us cheaper meat.

Growth hormones are generally implanted behind the animal's ear, added to feed, or placed in a doping mix for animals being fattened in feedlots prior to slaughter. A withholding period is required prior to the animal's slaughter to cleanse its system. The USDA/FSIS randomly checks animals in the slaughterhouse and tests for HGP residues. The CFIA takes similar monitoring actions. Are these measures enough to make the beef safe?

HGP use has been ongoing in North America for decades. However, Europe banned this practice long ago. In fact the EU is so strongly opposed that in 1989 the European Economic Community (EEC) banned the import of meat from hormone-treated cattle, thus cutting off most U.S. and Canadian beef exports to European countries. Other nations have taken similar action.

The public furor that resulted from lifting of this import ban against hormone-treated American beef in South Korea in 2008 shows how differently some nations feel about the issue. Thousands of Koreans protested in the streets, truckers threatened not to transport American beef, and there were boycotts of American beef and American restaurant chains such as McDonald's. This is a far cry from the current attitudes of most North Americans on the issue.

So, do HGPs threaten meat eaters' health? Agencies and governments, experts, and consumers disagree. Those on both sides of the issue argue that the other side's viewpoint has been influenced by special-interest groups, committees, and masquerading experts who really don't know what they are talking about. The USDA and FDA and other defenders of the practice say that HGPs are safe: that there is no hard evidence to prove any threats to human health; that many of the hormones in use (three out of six) are "natural"; that all is well as long as the hormones are administered properly. And that controls are in place to make sure there is no public health risk.

In the EU's view, the long-term effects of this practice on humans are still largely unknown, so we can't say whether it is safe or unsafe. The EU experts feel that scientific evidence is insufficient to form definitive conclusions either about the likely amounts of HGP residues remaining in treated meat, or what levels could be considered safe or toxic. The EU expert committee on HGPs has also concluded that the available evidence argues that risks could be very different at different stages of life: Those most at risk are prepubescent children. For women, the risk might exist right through menopause. We need more research on these issues.

The Consumer Federation of America, the Center for Science in the Public Interest, and other environmental, animal-rights, and consumer groups in the United States have long urged a ban on the use of growth hormones in American meat production. Even some people in the livestock production business (including ones with whom I have discussed this issue personally), point out that hormones are not always correctly administered, and accurate test results are difficult to obtain, resulting in questionable safety.

Many American consumers are concerned about the HGP issue. Some worry about a possible link between use of growth hormones and increased risk of breast, prostate, and colon cancer. The European experts agree that these risks potentially exist, along with developmental, immunological, neurobiological, immunotoxic, and genotoxic effects. (Don't expect me to spell all these out, but the broad categories certainly give us enough to worry about.) One concern that has been circulating for years among my friends is that such use of hormones could be to blame for the early onset of puberty that they are noticing among their children. They fear that this could lead to increased cancer risk later on in life. I have also found research that has linked beef eating among mothers—yes, among mothers—to decreased sperm count in their sons! These concerns are similar to those surrounding the use of hormones in milk cattle (see chapter 7).

Then there is the environmental dimension of the controversy. Critics of HGPs point to studies showing that growth hormones, excreted in cattle manure, can end up in our lakes and streams and in our fish. Some of the photographs of the deformed fish are hard to forget. As usual, defenders have a counterargument. They say hormone use aids the environment by reducing greenhouse gases.

After plowing through numerous research studies and expert group meeting reports, my personal opinion is that the Europeans are right. We still do not know enough about what all those "natural" (yes, and just as many synthetic) cattle growth hormones are doing to our body over the longer term. The practice could turn out to be a major risk . . . or it could turn out to be harmless. In the meantime, and while waiting for better hard data, we may wish to be cautious, particularly in the case of our children. If I knew then what I know now, I would not have given hormone-treated meat to my prepubescent child.

Unwanted Toxic Residues

THE USDA/FSIS-managed National Residue Program is failing to keep our beef safe from potentially harmful veterinary drug residues, chemical residues, and heavy metals. This is the conclusion of the U.S. Office of the Inspector General's (OIG) 2010 audit report of the program. The report is enough to turn anybody off eating meat.

One of the ways such toxic substances get into our beef (and other meats and poultry as well), is through drugs being added to feed for either preventive or therapeutic purposes (as in fish farming, which we looked at in the previous chapter). Because a "withdrawal" period is required between the times that animals are given antibiotics and they are slaughtered, antibiotic residues are probably not a major health issue in domestic meat and poultry. (However, I have read research that has found higher than FDA-allowed levels of a wide range of antibiotic residues in some imported meat and poultry products.) But no system is foolproof.

Reportedly, calves may get a particularly hefty dose of antibiotic if they are given "waste milk." This is milk from cows that have been given antibiotics. Such milk is not allowed to be sold for human use during a defined withdrawal period during which drug residues exit the cow's system (see page 195). Of course, producers are not supposed to bring their cattle or calves (or other animals) to the slaughterhouse while they have drugs in their system, because it can then get into our meat. But, as inspection reports show, it happens. The National Residue Program is meant to catch any producers that are breaking the rules. Inspectors at the slaughterhouses test the meat for veterinary drugs and then compare the test results with the established, so-called safe tolerance levels. But clearly all this is not enough. The inspector general's report concluded that even when unsafe levels of veterinary drugs are found in our meat, the meat is not being recalled.

Then there are all those agriculture and industry-caused toxic substances. According to the OIG report, meat is only being tested for one type of toxic pesticide residue. If this is so, it means that meat contaminated with residues of many synthetic pesticides and other toxic chemicals (including dangerous POPs, such as those we looked at in connection with seafood, and that also crop up in dairy products; see pages 9 and 196) will go into the marketplace for us to eat.

But drug residues and agricultural/industrial chemical residues, are not the only substances slipping through the testing net. Unlike other nations, the United States has apparently not established tolerances for potentially toxic heavy metals in meat, such as copper, arsenic, lead, and cadmium. This came to light in an embarrassing incident in 2008, when Mexico rejected a shipment of U.S. beef because the copper levels were above Mexico's tolerance levels. It turned out that the United States hadn't tested the meat for copper because it didn't even have a tolerance threshold for it. The same applies to arsenic and some other heavy metals that can turn up in beef. There *is* an established tolerance for arsenic in poultry (see page 149). The reason is that arsenic-containing drugs are commonly placed in the feed of chickens. However, the resultant chicken litter (including chicken "crap" and any spilled chicken feed, as well as feathers, dead insects, and rodents or whatever) is then nicely recycled into feed for feedlot cattle under our industrialized system of production. No one tests for arsenic in beef.

How dangerous are such usually small amounts of residue in our meats? Some of the drugs that are being found in beef (such as penicillin—yes, it has turned up in veal) can cause reactions in people who are allergic. In sufficient quantities, substances such as copper and arsenic can cause skin lesions, hypertension, kidney, and stomach or liver damage in humans (and who knows what else it can cause in children). We don't really know a great deal about how regular intake of small amounts in our food will affect us (see also discussion in connection with rice, page 255). Either way, we would prefer not to have them in our meat and poultry. Unfortunately, no amount of cooking will destroy such residues. In some instances, cooking will actually break them down into other substances that are even worse for us.

Imported meat and meat products are not safe from such toxic substances, either. Only a small percentage is caught by inspectors. Again, a lot of toxic substances are simply not being tested for. Let's look at an example. In 2010, inspectors found a shipment of corned beef and cooked beef from Brazil to contain unsafe levels of the potent antiparasitic drug Ivermectin. This drug is used for both animals and humans. But is not safe for everyone, and can sometimes damage the nervous system of sensitive people. Of course, the contaminated shipment of processed beef was refused entry. But—and this is where it gets worse—the USDA found that several other meat shipments from the same source (most likely, also similarly contaminated) had already entered the country and were in our food supply in the form of cooked canned and frozen beef products, under various popular labels. The suspect meat products were later identified and recalled—that is, the ones that hadn't already been eaten. All kinds of meat and poultry—be they domestic or imported—may carry residues of veterinary drugs, pesticides, and heavy metals. Unfortunately, we have no way of protecting ourselves against such residues, except through smart purchasing decisions. Maybe "know your cow" is the best strategy. But how often can you do that?

ARSENIC-LACED POULTRY?

With FDA approval, the broiler poultry industry (now no longer including Tyson) is giving its chickens and turkeys feed with added arsenic, to make them gain weight faster. These arsenic-containing drugs help to control parasites. As a bonus, the feed can also improve pigmentation. Usually organic arsenic is involved, which is not as toxic to humans as the **inorganic** version is. (However, there is now some evidence that argues that the organic arsenic converts into the more toxic inorganic arsenic when it combines with bacteria in the chicken or turkey manure—which is what we will have in our fertilizer, and, in cattle feed, if it contains poultry litter.) We spend so much money trying to get arsenic out of our water supply, and here we are, adding it to our food!

This practice is not allowed in organic poultry feed, and such arsenic-based food additives are also banned in Europe and many other countries. In December 2009, the Center for Food Safety and the Institute for Agriculture and Trade Policy jointly filed a petition with the FDA to remove arsenic from animal feed. Testing has come up with different kinds of conclusions about how much of this arsenic residue remains in the muscle meat or livers of chickens. Of course, the chicken livers have more, but with considerable variation from chicken to chicken. No wonder, as the Institute for Agriculture and Trade Policy has pointed out, quantities given to poultry are not strictly controlled. Who knows how much some of them are getting? In a few cases the levels may be enough to cause neurological problems in children or adults who eat a lot of chicken livers regularly. Naturally, the National Chicken Council says there's no problem. What would you expect?

Are Preservatives in Deli Meat Worth a Thought?

DELI MEATS ARE the most popular deli item in America. We eat a lot of ready-to-eat products such as hot dogs, ham, corned beef, roast beef, pastrami, and turkey, in addition to the many kinds of sausage that are on the market (see sidebar, page 134). Deli meats are convenient: great for a sandwich or a snack, requiring little or no cooking.

From a nutritional perspective, many deli meats have a high fat and salt content. From a safety perspective, there is the risk of *Listeria* bacteria and the issue of sodium nitrite, normally used as a preservative and color fixative. It is the nitrite preservatives in such deli items as hot dogs that give them that pretty pink appearance and great taste. Who would want to eat hot dogs if they were a dreary gray? Adding sodium nitrite also slows down spoilage and extends the shelf life of deli meats. As usual, there is a positive spin to a risky practice.

THE PATRIOTIC BUT UNHEALTHY HOT DOG

Humphrey Bogart is reported to have said, "A hot dog at the ballpark is better than steak at the Ritz." A lot of people would agree with him. Frankfurters, or "dachshund sausages" as they were apparently originally called, are a very popular example of deli meats. Most Americans, including children, eat them regularly. Eating hot dogs is almost a patriotic act: It is estimated that, about seven billion hot dogs are consumed in the United States between Memorial and Labor days, and about twenty million hot dogs annually. Yes, it's true—there is even a National Hot Dog [and Sausage] Council.

Consumer Reports has called hot dogs "tidy little bundles, of sodium, additives, and fats." In the United States, except in the case of soy hot dogs, they are made of beef, poultry, pork, or a combination of these, plus water, salt, seasonings, and often nonfat milk or cereal. At least, thanks to USDA regulations, frankfurters now contain no more than 30 percent fat. But they are loaded with nitrites. Some studies have linked hot dogs to childhood cancer—either when eaten in large quantities by young children, by women during pregnancy, or even by the children's fathers. Such findings still need to be confirmed.

Hot dogs may also carry bacteria such as *Listeria monocytogenes,* which are so dangerous for pregnant women. Growth of these bacteria is not completely prevented by sodium nitrite or by refrigeration. Although labeled "fully cooked," hot dogs are best treated like raw meat in terms of storing, handling, and thorough heating. They should not be eaten to excess—even at the ballpark.

Nitrites also have a negative side. It is generally accepted that, in large enough quantities, nitrites could damage your health over the longer term. Some studies suggest that nitrites from food may increase the risk of cancer (of the colon, stomach, pancreas—and perhaps even of the oral cavity, bladder, and esophagus) and serious lung disease, as well as trigger migraine headaches. The amounts of processed meat products used in several of these research studies has been frighteningly small by American meat-eating standards. Research also shows that infants are particularly susceptible to these compounds because of their lower body weight and their underdeveloped enzyme system. In worst-case scenarios, nitrites have been linked to brain tumors in infants and leukemia in children. Animal studies, as well as some documented human cases, argue for mothers-to-be and nursing mothers to limit their intake of nitrite-containing foods.

But is there enough in our deli meat to hurt us? The meat industry says there isn't. The FDA has set limits on the levels of nitrite that can be used in American processed foods. Deli meats now contain much less than they did ten or twenty years ago. Some industry statements claim that nitrite levels have dropped by as much as 80 percent since the 1970s. The meat industry also tells us that not only is any sodium nitrite used in "tiny" amounts, but it is, after all, a "natural substance." (Natural is always good, right? But then, arsenic is also natural. . . .) Besides, only a small percentage of the nitrite we get originates in meat. We may be getting more from certain *nitrate*-containing vegetables (nitrates can potentially convert into nitrites) and even from our own saliva.

The bottom line: After all these decades of nitrite use, and all the studies done, a lot of questions still remain concerning the extent of our risk from eating nitrite-processed meats. So, what can we do? Let's face it, most of us would find it very difficult to give up deli meat. But some of us eat too much of it every day and feed too much of it to our children. People with a high food-risk rating, and those responsible for what young children eat, may want to take it easy on deli meats.

Say No to "Mad Cow" Beef

MAD COW DISEASE (more correctly, bovine spongiform encephalopathy, or **BSE**) is definitely something we don't want. BSE has been called an "emerging crisis" in food safety. Researchers now believe it dates as far back as the 1970s, and may have actually spread from sheep to cattle (through feeding cattle meat-and-bone meal that contained infected materials from the sheep). We did not hear much about BSE until the epidemic in the United Kingdom in 1992–1993.

BSE is a fatal neurological disease of cattle, rare but very dangerous. Strictly speaking, humans can't get mad cow disease. What we can get is a human variant of the disease called **Creutzfeldt-Jacob disease (CJD)**. CJD can also have other causes than infected food. This is an incurable brain disease, believed to be caused by abnormal and vicious forms of protein called **prions**. Prions apparently bore numerous microscopic holes into the brain, which lead to hallucinations, dementia, and death. It seems incredible, but the time period between infection with prions and appearance of first symptoms can be as long as seven years, and occasionally even as long as sixteen years (similar to leprosy).

Most people don't realize that animals other than cattle can also carry prion-caused diseases similar to BSE, such as scrapie and chronic wasting disease. Such animals include sheep, deer, elk, and mink. Even less is known about our risk from these diseases, but there are suspicions. In fact, in February 2009, a Texas company did recall elk meat because the elk may have had chronic wasting disease.

Yes, there have been BSE-infected cows both in Canada and the United States. In Canada (at time of writing), eighteen cases have been confirmed, including one in February 2010 in Alberta. The Canadian beef industry has suffered as a result, with a temporary bans on Canadian cattle crossing the Canadian-U.S. border. Up until 2010, three BSE-infected cattle had also been found in the United States (in Alabama, Washington, and Texas). One of these cattle had been born in Canada. These BSE incidents had a disastrous effect on U.S. beef exports. In one of these cases, the meat actually entered the U.S. food supply but was quickly caught. That is the official story. But the Congressional Research Service (CRS) briefing of U.S. Congress in January 2005 acknowledged that in actual fact some of the thirty-eight thousand pounds of recalled meat (which was not from only the suspect cow, but from some twenty others that were at the slaughterhouse the same day that just might also have been infected) had already been eaten prior to the recall. Other rumored incidents of BSE in cattle are around, including a mysterious case where the brains and spinal cords of two cows reportedly went missing, so that they could not be tested. Who knows if such stories are true or not.

There have also been at least three cases of the human disease, CJD, in the United States. All were believed to have been caused by eating BSE-contaminated beef while overseas. One woman apparently acquired it in Great Britain, the country worst affected, before moving to the United States (the public health officials wished she had stayed there). Another victim was probably infected in Saudi Arabia as a child. The third moved between Great Britain and Texas and probably caught it while he was out of the country.

Both the U.S. and Canadian regulators assure us that we can now safely eat meat without worrying about CJD. The two countries are harmonizing new safety measures to protect cattle and consumers. The focus in the United States is on preventing BSE from entering the country and to prevent it from spreading if it does enter. Measures include import bans, feed restrictions, and animal testing. Stricter rules have been issued to slaughter facilities and rendering firms, but it has taken time for all the large and small facilities to comply.

Considerable attention has been given to the issue of cattle feed to prevent the spread of the disease among animals. When BSE first turned up it sent a shock wave around the world. We suddenly became aware of the practice of "cattle cannibalism." BSE spreads by the feeding of infected body parts and blood of dead cattle to live cattle. To make our food (and cosmetics) safer, the government has banned use in cattle feed of those parts of dead cattle that carry the highest risk of BSE—mainly brains and spinal cords from older cattle. This was believed to make our food animals about 90 percent safe from BSE. Critics (including members of U.S. Congress) pointed out that such risky materials were still allowed in other animal feed (such as pork feed and pet food) and mix-ups do occasionally occur at feed mills. This led to the passage in 2009 of "enhanced" regulations that prohibit such risky materials from being used anywhere in the animal feed system (Fido is now safer, too). This had already been the law in Canada since July 2007.

But are such regulations always complied with? I reviewed the latest FDA and state inspection reports of domestic facilities. According to these, most companies are indeed complying. At the same time, inspections at our ports are still finding imported meat products that contain the riskiest animal body parts. (How many are not being caught by inspectors?). We may still feel safer eating **grass-fed**, organic, or kosher meat. Some experts point out that kosher laws are stricter than government standards, and provide extra measures of protection by eliminating older and even slightly sick cattle (as well as other animals and poultry) from the food supply. The method of killing may also be less likely to scatter potentially dangerous brain matter. During the height of the "mad cow" scare, a Los Angeles kosher supermarket owner put up a bright yellow and red banner in front of his store. It read: DON'T GET "MAD" GET KOSHER / KOSHER MEAT IS SAFE. The sign brought in new customers and reassured existing ones.

The chances are that BSE will not become a major food safety issue in North America. But we can never be sure. The fact that outbreaks in cattle in Canada still seem to be occurring as this book goes to press is a worry. But at least they seem to be caught. Measures in recent years *have* generally made our beef safer—at least from the BSE perspective. However, should BSE spread to North America, remember that steaks and roasts are the safest cuts of beef to eat. Avoid deli meats, sausages, and ground beef (as these are likely to contain meat scraped off the spine—the most dangerous part of a diseased cow). If you must eat ground meat, consider organic, grass-fed, or kosher—or buy muscle meat and have it ground up right in front of you, to make sure that is all it contains. Remember, cooking, drying, or freezing BSE-infected meat will not make it less dangerous.

Bird Flu Is Still Flying Around

MANY OF US are also worried about **avian influenza**, commonly known as "bird flu," and wondering if we can get it from our food. However, we are less concerned about this disease now than we were a few years ago when it was receiving more news coverage. But believe me, it's still around.

Avian influenza is caused by type A strain of the influenza virus (H5N1 virus). Relatively few humans have ever caught bird flu— an estimated five hundred cases were confirmed by WHO as of July 2010. The reason avian influenza is so frightening is the over 50 percent fatality rate (300 of the 505 WHO–confirmed cases as of August 31, 2010 have proven fatal).

The symptoms of avian influenza can easily be mistaken for ordinary seasonal flu, although it is much more dangerous: high fever, sore throat, cough, muscle aches as well as chest pain, difficulty in breathing, a hoarse voice, sometimes bloody sputum, watery diarrhea without blood, abdominal pain, and vomiting. Other kinds of symptoms such as eye infections and bleeding nose and gums occur in certain cases. At some point pneumonia usually develops. However, in a few instances of infection there have been no respiratory symptoms at all.

Bird flu has now spread to many countries. Nor is it any longer just for birds. Cases have been reported in swine, cats, dogs, stone martens, and even tigers and leopards, as well as in humans. It has now turned up not only chickens but also in several kinds of birds we eat, including turkeys, quails, ducks, geese, and guinea fowl, as well as in pet birds and wild birds. In spite of control efforts, outbreaks are continuing in Asia, Africa, the Middle East, and Europe. Just in the first four months of 2010, eleven countries around the world reported outbreaks in domestic poultry or wild birds or animals. It is suspected that wild birds, which usually do not show any symptoms and which may traverse great distances, are responsible for much of the spread of the disease. There are also other ways the virus can spread from farm to farm. In some countries, such as Egypt, bird flu is considered endemic. Avian influenza is not over yet. The virus that causes it is still evolving and becoming increasingly contagious. There are fears that the Asian version of the H5N1 virus will eventually become adapted to humans and result in a huge human pandemic. One of the prevention problems is that domestic birds like ducks may become infected without showing any symptoms. Researchers are looking closely at clusters of illnesses among humans to assess the likelihood of human-to-human transmission.

What many Americans don't know is that in September 2008, a case of one of the milder strains of avian influenza was identified in a pheasant on an Idaho game farm. The initial report sent to the World Organization for Animal Health (OIE) estimated that potentially some thirty thousand birds might be "at risk."

Can you get avian influenza from eating poultry? Contrary to what is often believed, most of the infected people have *not* contracted this virus from eating virus-contaminated poultry or eggs. They have caught it as a result of *touching* H5N1-infected live or dead birds (usually chickens, turkeys, or ducks), or from contact with surfaces or objects that are contaminated by the feces or saliva of infected birds during slaughter, defeathering, food preparation, or the cleaning of pens where birds are kept. Many cases of the disease have occurred in children, who are often given the chore of cleaning the bird pens on family farms. The virus may also be caught by inhaling contaminated dust. However, undercooked chicken could be risky: WHO *has* recorded a few cases linked to consumption of dishes containing raw poultry blood.

Overall, it is safer to avoid eating H5NI-contaminated poultry and poultry products. That applies not only to chickens, but also to other food birds (and to leopards and tigers!). The virus is very contagious and is not killed by refrigeration or freezing. It can survive for a month or more in a refrigerated environment.

THE REAL STORY ABOUT SWINE FLU

Things were bad enough when Americans were afraid of getting bird flu or the human version of mad cow disease. Then, starting in April 2009, it was pork's turn. News of an outbreak of "swine flu" spread around the world. Americans became afraid of eating pork and any food using that "other white meat" as an ingredient. The value of shares in meat companies fell. Because there had been several cases of swine flu in the United States, several other countries banned U.S. pork imports. Those in the pork business were afraid that even more would opt out. Actually, swine flu is not new. The *real* swine flu is a common respiratory disease of pigs, caused by a strain of the influenza virus. Reportedly, over 51 percent of pigs in the north-central United States show signs of having had the infection at some time or other. (You have never seen a pig sneeze or cough? Look again, next time you visit that farm fair—but keep your distance.) Until 2009, there had been quite a few cases of *human* flu (and also of bird flu) in pigs, but few cases of swine flu in humans— only about one a year. These few cases of "human" swine flu had been the result of *direct* contact between pigs and people, mainly among swine farmworkers and children at fairs. There had also been at least one short-lived mysterious outbreak of swine flu among soldiers at Fort Dix, back in 1976 (when four soldiers became ill and one died). But the 2009 outbreak was much worse.

The truth was that in 2009, people were giving swine flu to one another, without the mediation of pigs or pork. It was not really swine flu but a hybrid virus. The swine flu virus had performed a genetic swap with other flu viruses. But the media kept calling it "swine flu" in spite of experts' and the government's efforts to rename it.

The FDA and CDC assured consumers that we could not get this flu from eating pork or pork products. What we call "swine flu" is no more a food safety issue than is a seasonal flu or a cold. It is spread person-to-person, usually when an infected individual sneezes or coughs, or when the virus lands on a surface that we touch and then transfer to our mouth. We are more likely to get it from a stair banister, a door handle, or someone's hand than from food.

At restaurants, the same situation applies: If an infected restaurant worker sneezes on our food—or, our fork—and we then put it in our mouth . . . Interestingly, although the FDA and CDC did not admit it, it *is* quite possible for people to catch swine flu from their food— probably more often from their salad than their pork chop, because salad is likely to be more exposed to coughing restaurant workers. Tomato flu, anyone?

Is Irradiated Meat Good or Bad?

FEDERAL REGULATORS HAVE progressively widened their approval of irradiation technology for beef, pork, lamb, and poultry since the 1990s. The purpose has been to make meat safer to eat. As an example, in 1992 the FDA approved irradiation at low doses of raw, fresh or frozen packaged poultry, to reduce the chance of illness caused by bacteria such as *Salmonella* and *Campylobacter* if the poultry is eaten undercooked or is badly handled during preparation. You can easily recognize packages of irradiated chicken at the store because they carry the international radura symbol along with the statement, "treated with irradiation" or "treated by irradiation."

Two issues are important as regard irradiated meat. First, does irradiation make meat *safer to eat*, in terms of avoiding potentially dangerous microorganisms? Second, is irradiated meat *safe to eat*, in the sense that irradiation has not introduced some new toxic substance into our meat that could hurt us? This is not simply playing with semantics.

Let's consider the first question: At the approved doses for meat, irradiation does not wipe out *all* bacteria in it. Nor does it destroy prions (the proteins that have been associated with mad cow disease) or prevent later contamination by food handlers (which is believed to account for about 20 percent or so of all cases of meat contamination). One could therefore argue that it might be safer to cook the meat well than to use irradiation. Cooking should destroy bacteria and any parasites equally well, or even better—including most of those later contributions from food handlers, which irradiation would not deal with.

On the positive side, irradiation makes raw meat safer to handle. Just touching contaminated meat could put us at risk for bacteria such as the deadly *E. coli* O157:H7, which takes such small numbers to make us ill. Irradiated meat also reduces cross-contamination of other foods by meat, which is a common cause of food-borne illness. Irradiation would especially help to lower risks if bacteria- or parasite-contaminated meat is eaten undercooked. This could reduce meat-caused illnesses in places such as schools, nursing homes, and hospitals, where people are not only more vulnerable to start off with, but also more likely to be fed undercooked meat, because food is prepared in larger quantities and therefore more likely to heat unevenly.

As for the second issue—that of safety of irradiation itself—our government and the meat industry say that irradiated meat will not harm us, as they also say about irradiated produce and other foods. As usual, not everyone agrees. Although irradiated meat may well be safe to eat, if you feel strongly about avoiding it, look for the irradiation label (see page 82).

Read Those Labels

AN ENORMOUS VARIETY of labeling is done on our meat and poultry products. That is, if you can read the fine print. Some of these are useful from a safety viewpoint, some not. The following discussion of labels is specific to the United States; however, meat and poultry labeling in Canada is very similar.

Country of Origin Labeling (COOL)

Meat and poultry were covered in the second phase of the progressive implementation of COOL in the United States (see page 77). The law does not apply to all meat products. The reasons for such arbitrariness are hard to understand. I even consulted the USDA experts, and although they were extremely helpful, they were also mystified.

COOL does cover muscle cuts of raw meat (such as steaks and roasts), ground beef and veal, lamb, pork, and goat. Raw chicken is covered, but other poultry products, such as turkey, duck, and game birds, are not. Whereas fresh and frozen meat are covered by the legislation, the COOL labeling requirement does not extend to meat products such as ham, bacon, roast beef, or other meats that have undergone further processing. Also excluded are meats that have been combined with another food, such as a breaded veal cutlet.

For meat or poultry to be labeled "Product of the United States," it has to come from animals that were born, raised, and slaughtered here. If, for example, the cattle or pigs were actually born in

Canada and then imported into the United States for fattening and slaughter, then the label would have to read "Product of the United States and Canada." If a package contains the meat of cattle from several countries—as it could in the case of ground beef—then it may read something like "Product from the United States, Mexico, Canada, and Australia."

Passed and Inspected

A "Passed and Inspected by USDA" seal on meat or poultry means that the product was produced in line with federal regulations and "under federal oversight" (see figures 4–6). During inspection, the animal and its internal organs are checked to make sure there are no signs of disease. Raw and processed meat and poultry products have different USDA marks to show that inspection took place. The mark contains the federal inspection number of the facility that produced the product.

Inspection mark on raw beef, pork, lamb, and goat	Inspection mark on processed beef, pork, lamb, and goat	Inspection mark on raw and processed poultry
Figure 4	*Figure 5*	*Figure 6*

Product Grading

Grading has to do with the *quality* of the product, *not* its safety. Federal grading has existed in the United States since 1927, with some changes along the way. While inspection is required, quality grading of meat or poultry is voluntary and is paid for by meat producers. It is simply a marketing tool that provides an evaluation of such aspects as tenderness, juiciness, and flavor of the meat or poultry, based on such factors as carcass maturity, firmness, texture, meat color, and marbling.

Certified

The term *"certified"* on meat refers to quality, not safety. It simply means that the USDA's FSIS and the Agriculture Marketing Service have officially evaluated the product for class, grade, or other quality characteristics (e.g., "Certified Angus Beef"). It can also be used in association with the name of another organization responsible for the *"certification"* process, e.g., *"Prime Meat Company's Certified Beef."*

Product Dating

Unlike meat grading, product dating *is* relevant to safety, and something we should keep an eye on. U.S. federal regulations do not require product dating, but many stores and processors choose to date poultry and meat products. If a date is given, it has to show the month and day. The date most relevant to meat safety is the *expiration date*, which refers to the last date for using the product while it is still wholesome. The *use-by date* (sometimes with such variations as "best if used by" or "best if used before") is determined by the manufacturer or producer, and refers primarily to quality. It does not imply that a product will be unsafe after a certain date, but many of us prefer to use it as a guide anyway and to buy and eat or freeze a product before this date. A *sell-by date* suggests how long the store should offer the product for sale. Again, it is safer to purchase the product before this date and to eat or freeze it within a few days. However, in theory, you can buy meat on sale a day before, or at the "sell-by" date, as long as the meat is unspoiled and you cook it that same day. Never buy packaged meat or poultry products with a missing or obscured sell-by date.

No Hormones

A producer or processor can use the terms "no hormones added" or "no hormones administered" on the label of beef or lamb products, only if they have provided the USDA with all the necessary documentation to prove that absolutely no hormones have been given to the cattle. The label is not approved for use on pork or poultry, unless it also states, "Federal regulations prohibit the use of hormones in pork/poultry," as that is the case with pork or poultry.

No Antibiotics

The USDA allows the terms "*no antibiotics added*" or "no antibiotics used" or "raised without antibiotics" in meat or poultry product labeling, again only if the producer has adequately documented that the animals were raised completely without antibiotics. In practice, such labeling can become quite contentious. It has even led to a lawsuit between rival poultry companies (Tyson Foods and Perdue) because of differences in opinion about the definition of *antibiotic*.

Certified Organic

To be "certified organic," meat or poultry have to meet the USDA's NOP requirements. The organic label on meat and poultry is a green circular symbol (see page 78). *Organic* is a more precisely defined term than *natural*, because it requires compliance to federal regulations. The USDA has fairly strict standards for organic meat, as it does for other organic foods. The animals must be raised on organic feed (grains and grasses) and not given feed made from parts of other animals, but may be given certain vitamin and mineral supplements. Growth hormone stimulants or antibiotics are also not allowed. If an animal is sick and has to be treated with antibiotics, then it has to be taken out of the organic program. Organically raised cattle have to have access to pasture. In general, organic meat and poultry, as is the case for other organic foods, are also minimally processed with artificial ingredients or preservatives. Irradiation is not allowed. Imported organic meat and poultry products have to meet the same organic standards as domestic producers. Owing to increased production costs, organic meat is almost always more expensive.

Natural

Consumers often confuse the term *natural* with *organic* and think that the former has something to do with the way the animal was raised. It does not. Presently, the USDA simply defines *natural* as food that is "minimally *processed* and contains no artificial ingredients." Therefore, as pertains to meat or poultry, the label only guarantees that no artificial ingredients, such as flavorings, coloring ingredients, or chemical preservatives, have been added to the product *after* the animal was slaughtered. It does not mean anything in terms of how the animal(s) was raised. There is nothing to stop "natural" meat producers from using antibiotics. Nor are they required to use certified organic feed grains or pasture or to provide cows with access to pasture. Some ranchers are switching to the "natural" label because compliance with its requirements is less difficult and less costly, and many consumers don't differentiate.

Certified Humane and Animal Compassionate

Humane certification is not done by government agencies. There are several private programs that do this, usually linked to an animal welfare organization. A "certified humane" or

Figure 7

similar label on meat, poultry, eggs, or dairy products is an animal-welfare label, offering no food-safety guarantees. It simply means that farmers, producers, and processors made sure the animals were well treated in terms of such issues as food and water, space, shelter, and handling. At times, a similar certification also covers humane slaughtering procedures and forbids hormone use. (See figure 7, the Certified Humane label awarded by Humane Animal Farm Care, a national nonprofit organization.) There are differences of opinion as to whether the "humane" label has anything to do with safety. Some dismiss it as mainly a marketing strategy, whereas others argue that humane treatment also translates into a better-tasting and safer product. How much this is wishful thinking is difficult to say.

Another similar label used by one grocery store chain is "animal compassionate." But the precise meaning of "humane" or "compassionate" treatment is debatable. Even the animal activists can't agree. The advertisers' bucolic image of "happy cows" munching away in green pastures, singing or talking to one another, or of pigs in "hog heaven" may be quite far from the reality.

Grass- or Forage-Fed

According to the USDA, *grass-* or *forage-fed* means that that the cattle's food source during all their life (except for milk prior to weaning) has come from natural grazing. The animals are not allowed to be fed corn, soy, and other by-products generally used in U.S. livestock production. The USDA also states that such animals "must have continuous access to pasture during the growing season." As in the case of so-called free-range chickens (see following labeling term), in practice this condition is open to a variety of loose interpretations. But standards for the "grass-fed" label *are* progressively being strengthened.

Free-Range

Free-range or *free-roaming* simply means that the birds bearing such a label were not housed in cages. All the producer has to do to obtain this label is to demonstrate to the USDA/FSIS that the poultry has been allowed access to the outside for most of their lives. But the image that many consumers have of chickens running around the farmyard being chased by children is rarely true. Under this rather loose definition, birds can be kept in open-air barns, with often only a few minutes of access to the outside—and still qualify as "free range."

Mechanically Separated

Mechanically separated meat or poultry is a pastelike product that has been produced by forcing bones with attached edible tissue through a sieve or other mechanical device, under high pressure. The purpose is to get that last little bit of meat off the bone. The bones themselves are discarded. In 2004 as a result of BSE fears, restrictions were passed that banned mechanically separated beef from the human food supply (it can still be used in pet food). However, pork and poultry processed in this manner are permitted in human foods, but have to be labeled "Mechanically Separated Pork/Poultry." This meat or poultry paste is used in making such foods as chicken nuggets and hot dogs. (Now you know how they got so nice and tender.)

But What About . . . ?

How can I tell if meat or poultry is spoiled?

You can *sometimes* tell by its appearance and smell that meat or poultry is spoiled, meaning that it is unfit or unsafe to eat. But this is not always the case. Nor is an item that appears spoiled always dangerous. However, don't buy or eat meat or poultry that smells like ammonia or sulfur (or has a cloyingly sweet smell), has changed in color (with areas of brown, gray, black, or green), or looks slimy or sticky. This rule applies to processed products such as sausages and cold cuts, as well as to fresh cuts of meat and ground meat. In such cases, the items could be tainted with dangerous microorganisms. Although thorough cooking might make such organisms harmless, the toxins and spores produced by certain bacteria can survive the cooking process. It is better to simply avoid the risk.

But meat and poultry can also change color as a result of improper freezing (whitish "freezer-burn"), or exposure to air. Although such items may taste like cardboard, they are not unsafe. Certain color differences are also normal. For example, ground meat will usually be red on the outside and grayish brown on the inside (because of lack of access to oxygen). When the outside starts turning brown, then it is likely that spoilage is beginning. Iridescent (rainbow) color on roast beef, lunch beef, or ham is a sign of oxidation, not spoilage. Certain odd smells are also harmless. When meat has been placed too close to onions, it can catch the odor.

Remember, meat or poultry may be "spoiled" in the sense of contaminated by bacteria, yet look and smell perfectly fine. What this means is that you cannot rely entirely on appearance and odor.

Why does packaged red meat stay pink for such a long time?

Pink meat is one of the tricks of the industry. An ingredient can be added to the meat, or packaging can be used to stabilize its natural red color pigment. The use of carbon monoxide is an example of this type of technology. When the package is opened, the gas escapes into the air (No, it will not hurt us). Other ingredients that help to maintain the red color are sodium ascorbate, rosemary extract, and citric acid. Unlike carbon monoxide, these ingredients actually become part of the meat product. The FDA and FSIS review any such new technologies to make sure they are safe as well as effective. It has been argued that slowing down the color change in meat can be dangerous since a change in color can warn people that the meat is spoiled.

Does the color of raw chicken have safety significance?

No, the color of the chicken skin varies from a creamy-white to yellow, depending on what the chicken has been fed. It has nothing to do with safety, nutritional value, flavor, or tenderness. Certain drugs given to poultry can also affect the skin and meat color of the birds.

Does a pink color in cooked meat or poultry mean that it is not done?

No, not necessarily, although it is often assumed that pinkness signifies rawness. The meat of smoked turkey you buy in a store is always a type of pink because of chemical changes that have taken place during smoking. In the case of poultry, even when safely cooked, it can vary in color from white to pink to tan. Younger birds often show the most pink meat. Poultry that is grilled or smoked outdoors can also show more pink color. Fresh pork and hamburgers can also still be pink after cooking to 160°F or higher. Only a food thermometer can accurately tell if the meat is adequately cooked, and almost all safety experts advise its use.

Which type of beef is safest for young children to eat?

Food-borne illnesses are a particularly serious risk for children under the age of five. Slightly contaminated food that may barely affect their parents can become a life threat to them. There are two kinds of meat you may want to think carefully about in the case of young children: ground meat and deli meats. Ground meat is particularly risky when eaten as hamburgers, more so if eaten out (as in fast-food restaurants) or when partially prepared ground meat products—such as frozen hamburgers—are cooked in a microwave. The problem, of course, is that in North America children begin to love hamburgers from an early age, and the fast-food industry does a very good job of marketing to them. Hamburgers are also cheap and quick for busy mothers to prepare at home.

If you can go to the trouble and expense, the safest approach is to buy muscle meat and grind it yourself at home—which hardly anyone does anymore. The next best thing is to buy a piece of sirloin or chuck steak and watch the butcher grind it up while you wait (and make sure he is wearing disposable gloves as he does so). At home, make sure the meat is well cooked. If this is done, cooked ground meat is normally just as safe from contaminant bacteria and parasites as muscle meat is. It is best to not give your young children much deli meat (including hot dogs) or bacon, unless clearly labeled "nitrite free," "low nitrite," or something similar, and such products should also be well cooked. Never feed your child a frankfurter right out of the package, even if labeled "fully cooked," without fully cooking it. Of course, they will be likely to eat the occasional hot dog or ham sandwich at their friends' place, but that is not enough to worry about.

How should frozen meat be safely defrosted?

Frozen meat (like frozen fish—see previous chapter) should be defrosted in the refrigerator—not at room temperature. If you need a faster defrost, do it in the microwave, or put it in a sealed bag, in a bowl of water, and keep changing the water frequently. Cook the meat as soon as it is defrosted. Make sure you place a dish under any defrosting meat, so that liquids do not leak and contaminate other foods or counters.

Is it safe to microwave hamburgers?

In theory, yes, microwaving hamburgers can be safe. But people often forget that some microwaves do not cook food evenly, and do not allow for this. Covering the hamburger and turning it over halfway through will make microwaving it safer. When finished, the hamburger should also be allowed to stand for a minute or two to finish cooking. The internal temperature should be at 160°F.

Is grass-fed beef safer?

It has been argued that grass-fed beef not only is leaner, and with some nutritional advantages, but is also safer. The USDA Organic Program's "Eat-Well Guide" makes this argument. It hints that grass-fed beef may have less *E. coli* and other disease-causing bacteria. There may also be other safety advantages—but at the moment, unproven. Such cattle do not consume feed that contains parts of other animals and are not as likely to be exposed to toxic chemicals or high levels of toxic molds or chemicals from low-quality grains or toxin-contaminated feed (for instance, feed containing arsenic-contaminated poultry waste). However, they may still ingest toxic substances from contaminated grass. The small percentage of ranchers who practice this approach argue that the animals are also happier, which certainly seems obvious. Some of us can also notice the difference in taste, particularly with beef.

Smart Ways to Reduce Your Risks

NORTH AMERICANS HAVE traditionally loved and trusted their meat and poultry. But in recent years some bestselling books, films, and news media reports have made us see our meat differently. It has been a wake-up call that has forced us to think about what we are eating. Actually, our meat is now much safer than it used to be. More controls are in place on meat producers and processors. Even slaughterhouses are more sanitary and better regulated. There are lower levels of nitrites in deli meats, and country-of-origin labeling on many of our meat products gives us a choice. Further improvements are presently being made, both in the United States and in Canada. But these still fall short of making our meat *completely* safe to eat. Unfortunately, our favorite meat and meat dishes also tend to be the riskiest: ground meat dishes, rare or medium-rare steaks, and deli meats. Ultimately, much of the safety of the meat we eat will be up to us. It will depend on decisions we make in the store, when we are preparing meat, and when we eat it, whether at home or when eating out.

Buy meat carefully. If buying fresh meat or poultry, purchase it from a reliable retailer. This is most important in the case of ground meat that is made, repackaged, or modified on the premises. Make sure to check the appearance, smell, and the date of any meat you buy to ensure it not spoiled (see pages 166–167). But remember that color in itself is not always an accurate indicator, and can be affected by factors other than spoilage. However, if the color of fresh meat is lighter or darker than usual, or the meat has an off smell or is slimy to touch, avoid it. Don't assume that meat in higher-end stores is always unspoiled. In recent months I have spotted outdated and badly spoiled nitrite-free luncheon meat, ditto a fresh leg of imported lamb—both at highly respected food stores. If buying frozen meat or poultry, make sure you get it from the deepest section closest to the cold. Remember that ground meat (beef, chicken, turkey, pork, and lamb) is the most dangerous kind of meat to buy, but much less so if made from muscle meat. If you can afford it, and are worried about hormones in meat or antibiotic-resistant bacteria, buy only meat and poultry labeled "hormone-free" or "organic."

Store correctly. The length of time you can keep meat and poultry varies by the kind and whether you keep it in the refrigerator or freezer. Generally speaking, meat and poultry should be stored in the coldest part of the refrigerator (as in the meat tray), separate from the foods you eat raw, such as salads. If you have leakage in your meat tray from a package of meat or poultry, wash the whole tray well with soap and water immediately, rinsing several times. The following chart is based on several USAID/FSIS sources.

STORAGE TIMES FOR REFRIGERATED MEAT

Note: If the product has no "use-by date" then it should be cooked or frozen before these times.

FRESH MEAT AND POULTRY

Steaks, chops, roasts (from beef, pork, lamb, and veal)	3–5 days
Chicken or turkey (whole or parts)	1–2 days
Variety meats (liver, kidneys, tongue, brain, giblets, and heart)	1–2 days
Ground beef, turkey, veal, pork, and lamb, and stew meats	1–2 days

HOT DOGS AND LUNCHEON MEATS

Hot dogs	Unopened, 2 weeks Opened, 1 week
Luncheon meats	Unopened, 2 weeks Opened, 3–5 days

DELI AND VACUUM-PACKED PRODUCTS

Store-prepared (or homemade) chicken, ham, and similar meats	3–5 days
Prestuffed pork, lamb chops, and chicken breasts	1 day
Store-cooked dinners and entrées with meat	3–4 days
Commercial brand vacuum-packed dinners with/USDA seal	Unopened, 2 weeks

HAM AND CORNED BEEF

Ham, canned, labeled "Keep Refrigerated"	Unopened, 6–9 months Opened, 3–5 days
Ham, fully cooked	Whole,1 week Half, 3–5 days Slices, 3–4 days
Corned beef in pouch with pickling juices	5–7 days

BACON AND SAUSAGE	
Bacon	1 week
Sausage, raw from meat or poultry	1–2 days
Smoked breakfast links, patties	7 days
Summer sausage labeled "Keep Refrigerated"	Unopened, 3 months Opened, 3 weeks
Hard sausage (such as pepperoni)	2-3 weeks
COOKED MEAT, POULTRY, AND LEFTOVERS	
Pieces and cooked casseroles	3–4 days
Gravy and broth, patties, and nuggets	1–2 days
Soups and stews	3–4 days

Prepare meat and poultry cautiously. Make sure that there is no cross-contamination between raw meat and other foods or surfaces. Fluid from deli products, such as hot dogs, should not be allowed to leak onto countertops, cutting boards, or touch other foods. (I always open packages in the kitchen sink and run the tap afterward.) When preparing hamburgers or other types of ground meat dishes that you need to handle, be extra careful to touch the meat as little as possible (try doing it with kitchen tools or disposable gloves). Whole chickens or large roasts are best prepared in the sink (which is then washed immediately) or on a large tray (again, immediately washed) rather than on the countertop.

Cook thoroughly. Avoid rare or medium-rare meat or poultry, especially in the case of ground meat products. Most bacteria, parasites, and viruses are killed if meat and poultry are thoroughly cooked. No lunch or dinner is worth getting a superbug. Buy a meat thermometer and use it. The USDA/FSIS provides the following cooking guidance concerning minimum safe internal temperatures:

- Beef, veal, and lamb steaks; roasts; and chops—to 145°F
- All cuts of pork—to 160°F
- Ground beef, veal, and lamb—to 160°F
- All poultry—to 165°F (check the temperature at the thickest part of the breast and leg)
- Hot dogs, until steaming hot—to 165°F

As for cooking hamburgers, aim for a temperature of 165°F or higher, inserting a cooking thermometer into the thickest part. Even if you are not in a high-risk group, you would be wise to avoid rare or medium hamburgers. Although it gives you some idea, meat color is not necessarily a good indicator of it being thoroughly cooked. Be particularly careful if you are microwaving, barbecuing, or cooking food in large quantities (as tends to be done in restaurants and institutions), as it is more likely to result in uneven heating. And pass up the steak tartare—it's not worth the risk.

Limit your overall consumption of meats and even poultry. Most meat-eating Americans and Canadians eat too much meat. Restrict how much you consume by eating small helpings (a reasonable helping of meat or poultry is no larger than the size of your palm) and not eating meat every day. There are some great vegetarian and vegan dishes based on legumes or vegetables that your family can learn to love, as mine has.

Restrict your consumption of deli meats. Yes, they are safer now than they used to be, but whichever way we look at it, we can certainly not prove that deli meats are good for us. Avoid eating large amounts of those that contain nitrite preservatives, and avoid eating deli products every day. For example, eating three hot dogs a week is probably too much. To be safer—buy nitrite-free hot dogs and cold cuts that taste just the same, even though they may not look as pretty when they are raw. But be extra careful about spoilage.

Pregnant women need to take extra precautions. Pregnant women should view deli meats and foods such as refrigerated pâtés and meat spreads as especially risky (canned or shelf-stable pâtés are safer). The main reason is the risk of contracting *Listeriosis*. If you really want to eat such foods while pregnant, then cook them until they are steaming hot. Yes, even your RTE sliced turkey, roast beef, pastrami, and all those other great sandwich meats.

Watch what meat your children eat. Limit the quantities of meat you give them, and to be cautious, avoid giving prepubescent children hormone-fed meat until we have more information about long-term risks. You need to be extra cautious with those hamburgers and limit the amount of nitrite-preserved deli products such as hot dogs, especially for your younger children.

Be especially careful when eating out or traveling. It is best to avoid hamburgers or any "mystery meat" dishes unless you are sure they are thoroughly cooked, and to not eat meat or poultry in street stalls or cheap restaurants, especially in developing countries. (I have learned about such risks the hard way.) If you are worried about mad cow disease when traveling in countries where it is widespread, eat only muscle meat and avoid ready-to-eat ground beef products (such as hamburgers, hot dogs, taco fillings, luncheon meat, and sausages), no matter how thoroughly cooked.

7

Dairy

IS THERE ANY food with a healthier image than milk? We have all heard, "Milk is nature's food," "Milk is the perfect food," and "Milk is pure." But is it safe? True, dairy products used to be much more hazardous before pasteurization was invented. It was not unusual for people to die from drinking milk. In fact, it is believed that the death of Edsel Ford, the son of the auto magnate, was due to the brucellosis he caught from drinking raw milk, which his father had insisted on as a cure for his ulcers. (Personally, I prefer the version where he died of a broken heart.) These days, brucellosis in milk is not something you need to worry about, unless you are a fan of raw dairy. But other potential risks are turning up in our milk and other dairy foods—things like hormones, antibiotics, dioxins, and metals. Even rocket fuel.

. . .

What We Eat

WELCOME TO MODERN dairy. Forget the image of your glass of milk coming from a milk cow wandering peacefully among green hills. That poor cow may be lucky if it gets a mound of grass while it sticks out its tongue between the bars of its small, cramped stall. Besides, that glass of milk you are drinking is not "cow's milk." It is "*cows'* milk." It could have the milk of a hundred cows mixed into it. The same with other dairy products. Welcome again to our industrial food supply.

This is not to say that dairy isn't healthy, no matter how many dairy cattle contribute. Milk and other dairy products such as yogurt, cheeses, butter, cream, and ice cream are great sources of protein and vitamins, as well as calcium and magnesium. Health benefits of dairy foods are not limited to bone health. Eating dairy just may reduce your chances of getting all kinds of unpleasant diseases such as diabetes, breast cancer, colon cancer, and more. Modern technology has made milk and milk products even better than the original version—at least, so the industry tells us—with all kinds of extra health-boosting nutrients. And a confusing array of fat and taste choices.

Dietary guidelines recommend getting two to three cups of milk and other dairy products per day, although the best amount depends on our age, gender, and our physical activity. Although almost all North American homes consume milk and other dairy, the statistics show that neither Canadians nor Americans consume enough.

Our dairy preferences have also changed over the last few decades. Overall, we have shifted away from the richer products toward low-fat or nonfat ones. The organics—milk, yogurt, and other products—have also gained in popularity. We are eating less of some dairy foods, such as milk, and more of others than we used to. The greatest decrease in demand has been for whole milk, buttermilk, canned and dry milk, cottage cheese, and even ice cream. Our consumption of low-fat milk, cheeses, and yogurt has increased. Surprisingly, butter has stayed about the same (even before the Julia Child influence reasserted itself on our cooking). Our new loves in recent years have been Italian cheeses and those shredded or grated cheeses in convenient zippered plastic packages.

Since 1993, when USDA certified organic milk first appeared in supermarkets, we have started to buy a lot more organic dairy. These days, organic dairy is everywhere, and the big food labels have moved in, as they have with other organic foods. Some consumer groups and food policy institutes claim that several of these dairy producers with herds of thousands of cattle are bending the organic rules. Up until 2007, consumer demand for organic dairy grew at a rate of about 20 percent per year. Of course, as always, organic milk and other dairy foods cost more. As the recession deepened, consumers found it easy to save money by switching back to regular milk, cheeses, yogurt, and other dairy.

Overall, we have a huge range of dairy to choose from in the marketplace.

Milk

We not only have milk of various fat content but also milk with low- or reduced-lactose content, flavored milk, *Acidophilus* milk, and milk fortified with nutrients such as calcium, vitamins A and D, DHA (docosahexaenoic acid, a component of omega-3, along with EPA). You can also buy organic milk, evaporated milk, condensed milk, powdered milk, and more. A light aside: almost all the milk we drink is cow's milk, but if you want a change, you can buy goat's, sheep's, or even water buffalo's milk. You probably will not find yak's or reindeer's milk at your local supermarket (and I would not recommend either for its taste unless you are used to them). Unfortunately for those who are eagerly waiting, camel's milk sales are also running into some hurdles—maybe just as well, as camels are so difficult to milk.

From a safety point of view, we have two basic choices in milk and many other dairy products: raw and pasteurized. The very large majority of North Americans prefer the safer, pasteurized dairy products. But a small percentage loves that raw milk or other raw dairy. These are the people at most risk for many—but not all—dairy contaminants.

KNOW YOUR MILK

Pasteurized milk can be considered safe. It has been heat-treated by one of the standardized methods approved by the government. This reduces the number of microorganisms present to levels where they are unlikely to cause disease and it extends shelf life. There are several variations of pasteurization, including the original process called vat pasteurization, high-temperature short-time (HTST) pasteurization, higher-heat shorter time (HHST) pasteurization, and ultra pasteurization (UP). What works best depends on the type of milk product. The most common method of pasteurization in North America today is HTST pasteurization, which raises milk temperatures to at least 161°F, for a minimum of fifteen seconds, followed by rapid cooling. Various estimates suggest that 97 to 99 percent of the milk sold in the United States is pasteurized. Canada requires that all milk available for sale in Canada be pasteurized, although farmers are allowed to drink raw milk produced by their own cows (or goats).

Raw (unpasteurized) milk is often unsafe. It is more likely to contain microorganisms—both good and bad. In some parts of North America, the number of raw milk drinkers is reported to be growing.

Cheeses

As in the case of milk, the general trend in the United States has been toward eating more low-fat, reduced-fat and no-fat cheeses. Our favorites are no longer Swiss and Cheddar, but the lower- fat mozzarella cheese, which has experienced an amazing climb since 1987. Mozzarella is the "pizza cheese," and we love pizza.

KNOW YOUR CHEESES

Natural cheeses can be unripened (e.g., cottage cheese and cream cheese) or can be ripened by bacteria (e.g., Parmesan, Swiss, and Cheddar), or mold (e.g., blue cheese, Brie, and Roquefort). These bacteria and mold are not harmful to our health except for certain people with allergies. U.S. regulations require that only pasteurized dairy be used in cheese production (unless the cheese is aged; see below).

Raw milk cheeses are natural cheeses made from milk that, prior to setting the curd, has not been heated above the temperature of the milk when it came out of the cow (104°F).

Aged raw milk cheeses are raw cheeses that have been aged for sixty days or longer. Canada and the United States presently permit the sale of raw-milk cheeses *only* if they *are* aged, which makes them safer. The aging period helps to reduce the cheeses' bacteria count because they become drier and more acidic, which slows the germs' reproduction.

Processed cheeses and processed cheese spreads are made of lower-grade pasteurized natural cheeses—often several—usually with added emulsifiers, food coloring, flavorings, preservatives, and a number of other dairy (such as milk and whey) and nondairy ingredients. They are milder in flavor, and also softer than natural cheese, which tends to make them more attractive to children. These cheeses are often sold packaged and presliced.

Yogurt and Other Dairy

Other dairy foods that we eat in North America include ice cream, butter, cream, milk puddings, and sour cream. Ice cream remains a big favorite. But yogurt is gaining in popularity, with frozen yogurt capturing some of the ice cream market. Eat a frozen yogurt, and you can pretend you are really eating a healthy food instead of a fattening dessert (I use this convenient excuse all the time).

Yogurt has been around for thousands of years. Basically, it is fermented milk. The FDA defines yogurt as a product made with bacterial culture containing *Lactobacillus bulgaricus* and *Streptococcus thermophilus*. Americans are now eating more and more yogurt, much of it coming from Europe. The industry is responding with an ever-growing variety of choices. The fact that the biologist Ilya Mechnikov theorized that *Lactobacillus* bacteria in yogurt can extend our life span doesn't hurt our craving for it, either. Nor does the fact that yogurt is often marketed as a cure for digestive problems, which plague plenty of us. Of course, yogurt was a lot healthier before we started messing around with it, adding flavors and colorings.

We can think of yogurt as falling into two groups: yogurt with significant numbers of live and active bacteria (live cultures), and yogurt with few live bacteria, or virtually none (see sidebar).

KNOW YOUR YOGURT

Yogurt with live or "active" cultures is the more popular type of yogurt in Europe. To be labeled as such, bacteria have to be there is significant numbers when they reach consumers. In North America, commercial yogurt with live and active cultures starts off with pasteurized milk. Homemade yogurt is also made with live cultures. Even frozen yogurt can have live bacteria. It is frequently stated that the live cultures are good for digestion and for several of our other ills. There is some research to back this up. This yogurt tends to taste tart.

Yogurt without significant numbers of live cultures is the more popular type consumed in North America. This kind of yogurt also starts off with live bacteria. However, it is subsequently heated to high temperatures to extend shelf life and to reduce the tart taste of the yogurt, also destroying most live bacterial cultures in the process. Yogurt products that do *not* contain live and active "good" bacteria include heat-treated yogurt, as well as such products as yogurt salad dressing, spreads that contain yogurt, yogurt-covered pretzels, and yogurt-covered candy.

Milk-Derived Ingredients

The food industry uses milk-derived ingredients in a wide variety of processed foods. These include baked goods, dairy desserts, snacks, drink mixes, soups, and many ready-to-eat meat and poultry products such as cooked sausages, breaded chicken (and chicken nuggets), meatballs, meat and poultry wrapped in dough, and pizza and calzones.

Such milk-derived ingredients include whole milk powder, nonfat milk powder, whey powder, lactose, and casein. These substances are often imported. After the melamine-associated scandals (see page 199), many American consumers began to view such imported milk-derived ingredients as an invisible threat in their foods. American dairy farmers aren't too happy about all these cheap imports, either.

Who Keeps It Safe?

OVER THE LAST few decades, milk production has become much more assembly-line in style and technologically advanced. There have been large increases in the number of dairy cows in North America and in the milk produced per cow. Changes have also occurred in the way that cows are treated and dairy is processed. There have been parallel changes in dairy imports. Such shifts in the industry have resulted in new safety issues and new challenges for our food regulators.

At the national level, the FDA, in collaboration with the states and other federal-level agencies, is in charge of ensuring the safety of both U.S. domestic and imported dairy products. Among the safety-oriented activities that are carried out (as much as resources allow) are inspecting production facilities and warehouses; working with and educating the milk industry on good sanitation practices; reviewing the safety of any additives used in dairy products;

monitoring safety of dairy animal feeds; and checking to make sure that any veterinary drugs used harm neither the cattle nor the dairy consumer. The FDA develops model codes, ordinances, and guidelines for dairy products and works with states to implement them. Much of the hands-on inspection, as usual, is carried out by the state agencies.

Raw dairy receives special attention. Our safety regulators are not happy that some people drink raw milk or eat raw cheeses. They don't like the problems that outbreaks create. If you think you want more good bacteria, eat a pasteurized probiotic yogurt or pop a capsule instead. Federal agencies in both the United States and in Canada have issued strong warnings against unpasteurized dairy. The usual position is that any benefits it might have are far outweighed by the health risks. States in United States vary in terms of whether they allow any raw milk sale, and in what form. Many are clamping down on the practice. At time of writing, only ten states permit retail store sales of raw dairy products. In a few, you are allowed to buy it directly from dairies, and sometimes at farmers' markets. In others (such as California) the regulations and safety standards established for sale of raw milk make it very difficult for farmers to comply—another way of restricting the practice.

The Big Choice in Dairy

DAIRY FOODS PROVIDE a good illustration of "good bugs/bad bugs" and of "good molds/bad molds." As noted, some bacteria and molds are essential for making delicious cheeses and fermented dairy products such as yogurt. Other unwanted ones can get in and can make us ill.

If you drink raw milk or eat other unpasteurized dairy foods, you are basically gambling with your health. Once again, as with produce, fish, and meat, raw (unpasteurized) milk, raw cheeses and other unpasteurized dairy foods are risky. But if you don't consume unpasteurized dairy, you don't need to worry as much about bacteria in dairy foods. The facts are simple. Milk straight from the cow is not always "pure." Tests have shown that 2 to 25 percent of raw milk carries those nasty bugs we have met before, such as *Campylobacter, Escherichia coli, Listeria, Salmonella, Yersinia, Brucella* spp., *Mycobacterium bovis,* and *Coxiella burnetti.* I well remember at age eight being thrilled that I was finally allowed to milk a cow (by hand, which is very rare these days) but being told not to drink from the bucket before the milk was boiled. How does "pure" milk pick up contaminants? Unfortunately, it can happen quite easily. Bacteria can be present in, or on the udders of the cow, particularly if the cow has mastitis (an udder infection). Some studies show that mastitis is increasing as more dairy farmers give their cattle hormones to increase their milk production (see page 191). If good "cow hygiene" is practiced, you can reduce the numbers of the bacteria, but you cannot eliminate them completely.

Every year hundreds of people—maybe thousands, given the unreported cases—still become ill from drinking raw milk or eating raw milk cheeses. The cheeses are usually such kinds as *queso fresco*, raw-milk Brie, feta, or raw sheep's and goat's milk cheese. During a seven-year period (1998–2005), the CDC traced forty-five outbreaks to bacteria in unpasteurized milk or cheese. Raw dairy still seems to cause somewhere between six and ten outbreaks each year in the United States; 2010 was a particularly bad year.

Usually the victims of raw dairy are people who belong to certain ethnic groups (such as people of Hispanic origin) for whom it is a cultural tradition. Or they are dairy farmers (not just Mom and Dad, but also the kids) or farmworkers for whom raw milk products are convenient. Or they are just raw-milk enthusiasts from all walks of life who simply believe that raw milk has powerful enzymes and a lot of "good" bacteria their body needs. I know people who make enormous efforts to obtain raw milk and rave about the health benefits.

But even *pasteurized* milk or milk products can be contaminated by bacteria. It happens much less frequently. When it does happen, contamination usually occurs in the factory and tends to affect more people than the raw dairy outbreaks. One of the most widespread ingredient-linked outbreaks in the American food supply was associated with nonfat powdered milk (made by Plainview Milk Products). It was caused by *Salmonella*—a bacterium that tolerates dry conditions very well (see chapter 10). The problem was traced back to contaminated processing equipment. More than two hundred products across the United States and Canada had to be recalled, including packaged nonfat dry milk, cappuccino, cocoa, other hot drink mixes, gravy mixes, malted milk powders, breakfast drinks, weight-loss drinks, Greek yogurt, whey protein, powdered dietary supplements, cakes, oatmeal mixes, and dairy shake blends. Even Dunkin' Donuts hot chocolate and Dunkaccino drinks were part of the recall. Of course it is ironic—and sad—that some were "recovery" drinks, meant to improve health, which are normally consumed by people who are more vulnerable.

One kind of bacterium that commonly turns up in both raw and ready-to-eat dairy (probably originating in food handlers) is the dangerous *Listeria monocytogenes*. *Listeria* is especially common in raw soft cheeses. During just a three-month period in 2009, outbreaks averaged one a month, each involving a number of Mexican-style fresh cheese products from a different company. As we also observed in connection with deli meats, this bacterium is very hardy and can even grow in the refrigerator, where we tend to keep our dairy foods.

People with HIV/AIDS are almost three hundred times more likely to become seriously ill with this bacterium than are people with normal immune systems. In addition, the "beware" list includes newborns; people undergoing chemotherapy; those with diabetes, kidney disease, cancer; even people who are taking glucocorticosteroid medications, and pregnant women (see sidebar).

. . .

A VERY BAD BUG
FOR PREGNANT WOMEN

The bacterium *Listeria monocytogenes* is a frightening food hazard because of its unusually high fatality rate—21 to 25 percent. Each year, at least twenty-five hundred Americans become seriously ill with listeriosis, more than one fifth of whom die of it. Although this bacterium sometimes causes nothing more than a fairly mild illness, or even no symptoms at all, reportedly about half of the people who get it end up in the hospital. Various estimates suggest that up to 20 percent of the population of the United States may be walking around with this bacterium in their body yet not showing any symptoms. This means that you and I will know several of them, or maybe even be a carrier. There may be an even higher incidence of carriers among food-industry workers. This is not good news for those of us who eat the foods they touch.

Pregnant women are about twenty times more likely to get sick from listeriosis than is their neighbor or friend who is not pregnant. In fact, according to the CDC, *about one third of listeriosis cases occur during pregnancy*. The results can be miscarriage or stillbirth, premature delivery, or infection of the newborn. The disease rarely kills the expectant mother herself. If you want to read some really heartbreaking stories, Google the first-person accounts of such cases online. The only good news is that there does not seem to be any evidence of the disease affecting the next pregnancy.

Because they are much more likely to be seriously affected by one or other of the dangerous bacteria that can contaminate dairy foods, people in high-risk groups—such as pregnant women and others—should make sure they make smart dairy choices. The U.S. federal government's basic advice is as follows, adapted from the interagency Web site www.foodsafety.gov:

Okay to eat:
- *Pasteurized* milk or cream
- Hard cheeses such as Cheddar and extra-hard grating cheeses such as Parmesan

- Soft cheeses such as Brie and Camembert, blue-veined cheeses, and Mexican-style soft cheeses such as *queso fresco, panela, asadero,* and *queso blanco* made from *pasteurized* milk
- Processed cheeses
- Cream, cottage, and ricotta cheese made from *pasteurized* milk
- Yogurt made from *pasteurized* milk
- Pudding made from *pasteurized* milk
- Ice cream or frozen yogurt made from *pasteurized* milk

Unsafe to eat:
- *Unpasteurized* milk or cream
- Soft cheeses such as Brie and Camembert, and Mexican-style soft cheeses such as *queso fresco, panela, asadero,* and *queso blanco* made from *unpasteurized* milk
- Yogurt made from *unpasteurized* milk
- Pudding made from *unpasteurized* milk
- Ice cream or frozen yogurt made from *unpasteurized* milk

I cannot stress the dangers of unpasteurized dairy too strongly. If raw dairy is so dangerous, why is it still available? We asked the same question in connection with commercially sold raw (unpasteurized) juices back in the produce chapter. The answer is the same—because such foods have a loyal and strongly committed following, and there are always ways around restrictions. It is very tempting to risk it if you really believe that the good bacteria and enzymes in raw milk will boost your immune system, improve your arthritis or heart condition, alleviate those nasty allergies, and decrease asthma and lactose intolerance. I have even found claims that it can reduce wrinkles (better than Botox) and prolong your life. Of course, a few of these same claims are also made for regular milk, and even more often for yogurt and for cheese. But before you rush out to find raw milk, remember that the scientific basis for such claims is weak at best. And there is that downside factor of higher risks.

Raw-milk enthusiasts are finding ways to obtain what they want. Underground raw milk networks are being established in places like New York and Los Angeles. The media sometimes publicize such networks, leading to a proliferation of their use. In many parts of the country you can legally buy raw milk if it is labeled "pet food," as long as you are not turned off by the idea of eating dog or cat food. Still another way is to get raw milk in both Canada and the United States is through agreements such as barter, raw milk co-ops, herd sharing, cow boarding, and cow sharing (see sidebar), which may involve some exchange of cash yet are not technically illegal sales of raw milk. Apart from anything else, there is something very nice about the idea of having your own cow, even if you can't have it in your own backyard.

NO MORE COW SHARING

California produces more milk than any other state in the country. Most of it is pasteurized, but some of it is consumed raw. One California milk producer estimates that there are at least one hundred thousand Californians who drink raw milk every week. Others say the total is much less—closer to forty thousand. But what everyone does agree on is that the number of Californian raw milk drinkers is growing.

Because raw milk is increasingly difficult to get in California, those who want it are turning to such programs as herd sharing or cow sharing to circumvent government restrictions. It is not illegal in states like California to drink milk from your own cow any way you like. One way that cow sharing operates is that you lease "part" of a cow for a nominal sum such as twenty-five dollars. In exchange, you are allowed to get a certain amount of raw milk per week. Although there is a per-gallon charge, this is defined as copayment for the cow's "room and board" rather than payment for the milk. Some states allow cow sharing, some don't, and others simply do not have a position on the issue. The FDA is against this practice. The cow does not have a say.

There are dairies which have set up such arrangements and regretted it afterward. According to the *Los Angeles Times* and *Crescent*

City (CA) Daily Triplicate, one of them was a well-established family-owned organic dairy in Del Norte County in California. The cow-share program they set up was only a very small percentage of their dairy business. The dairy owners did all the right things. Before people could buy a cow share, they had to read a pamphlet about the dangers of drinking raw milk and sign an agreement stating that the dairy was not liable for any negative effects that resulted. This made it the consumers' decision and their risk.

Afterward, the dairy was very glad that it had those signed agreements. Unfortunately there was an outbreak of the *Campylobacter* in the milk, one of maybe a dozen or more cases in this one county of California in a six-month period in 2008. At least fifteen of these cow-share members became ill with the usual symptoms of stomach cramps, diarrhea, vomiting, and nausea. One woman became seriously ill, with nervous system complications and partial paralysis. Such complications are rare but occasionally do happen with infections caused by this bacterium. The dairy owners again acted responsibly, immediately alerting each of the cow-share owners even before they were positive that the dairy's milk was the cause.

After this incident the dairy stopped the cow-sharing program. That did not stop most of their customers from drinking raw milk. They just looked for another dairy.

Molds—As Always

As MENTIONED, DAIRY foods can contain both good and bad molds. The good ones contribute to Roquefort, Stilton, Gorgonzola, and other blue cheeses. The bad ones could make us sick if they spew out those dangerous mycotoxins we looked at in connection with fruits and vegetables (see page 54). It doesn't happen all the time, but it does occur. Heating the milk or other dairy food will do little to reduce the levels of such toxins.

How do such dangerous toxins get into our "pure" dairy foods? Usually they are there in the milk already, or enter soon after the cow is milked. A main source is mold-contaminated dairy cattle feed. Molds can enter grain crops (e.g., corn) while they grow or are in the process of being stored, and are then fed to cattle. This can occur in spite of the existing strict guidelines on such toxins in dairy cattle feed. In addition, testing of grains is difficult and not always accurate (see page 248). Or the molds get into poorly stored feed. The dairy cattle can eat such moldy food, complete with toxin, and produce milk contaminated with a mold toxin as quickly as twelve hours afterward. Dairy farmers in North America are very aware of this issue, but it is a much greater problem in some other countries.

These more dangerous molds can also enter dairy foods during processing or in our own homes, even though most of these foods are refrigerated. Even if the majority do not produce mycotoxins, any mold could set off mold allergies or give you respiratory problems. Entrance of molds during processing is frequently caused by poorly cleaned equipment, fungal spores floating around in the processing plant, or unsafe storage or transport. In our own kitchen, the causes are similar. What you would see are the fuzzy black, white, or green mold spores on the surface of your cheese, yogurt, or sour cream. What you don't see in moldy dairy (again, as with moldy fruit) are the roots or those toxins, which can spread much further, particularly in the case of a soft cheese or other soft dairy (don't just spoon away the spot). You may not always be able to see, smell, or taste the difference in the surrounding food. Fruit-containing yogurt may be contaminated through the fruit ingredient.

Even aflatoxin can turn up in our dairy foods. Aflatoxin is the most dangerous of the mycotoxins. That is, as far as we presently know (see pages 55 and 248). Reportedly Saddam Hussein even included aflatoxin in his biological weapons program. Certain aflatoxins are proven liver toxins and carcinogens. Some have been linked to the frightening, and at times fatal, Reye's syndrome, which affects all body organs, but especially the liver and brain. Children are especially vulnerable. In North America, we are not at risk for acute aflatoxicosis (unless the toxin is used as a suicide weapon, as happened in one recorded case—which pleased the researchers because it supplied them with considerable data on symptoms and effects). But we could be at risk for chronic exposure, which produces vague and difficult-to-diagnose symptoms. The aflatoxin that has occasionally turned up in dairy products such as fresh milk, nonfat dry milk, cheese, and yogurt is aflatoxin M1. It is not the worst, but is still possibly carcinogenic. Because of this, and the fact that vulnerable children consume so much milk, the U.S. government routinely monitors milk and milk products for aflatoxin contamination, to make sure that the levels stay below the established 0.5 parts per billion (ppb) action guideline.

It is difficult to say how well such preventive measures are working. In spite of the acknowledged importance of this issue, there seem to be relatively few recent and reliable studies of aflatoxin M1 levels in U.S. fluid milk, powdered milk, or other milk products.

A brief review of several studies suggests that this toxin is likely to be present in less than 2 percent of cases of moldy cheese. But still, for those of us that eat a cheese frequently, such risk is not to be dismissed. Very little is known about how much regular low levels of aflatoxin exposure from our food will affect our health. And let's remember, molds are everywhere. Whatever amount our milk or other dairy contains will add one little bit more to the total we are getting from all possible sources. This could just be the straw that broke the camel's back—or, the dose that ruined our liver.

The Forgotten Hormones

THE CHANCES ARE that if you live in the United States, much of the dairy that you consume is made of milk from hormone-treated cows. It is estimated that between 17 to 70 percent (USDA estimates are at the lower end) of U.S. dairy cows are injected with a hormone called recombinant bovine somatotropin (rBST), to increase milk production. This hormone was originally sold by

Monsanto under the brand name of Posilac. It is believed that by the time milk is pooled, *most* dairy products sold in the United States are likely to have at least some milk from rBST-treated cows. Should that worry us? Well, according to consumer surveys, we are less concerned now about hormones in milk than we were back in the 1990s. Maybe only around 10 to 15 percent of us are worried enough to actually change what milk or dairy we buy. Is that smart?

Posilac is a genetically engineered version of a natural hormone produced by cows. The FDA approved it in 1993. It has *not* been approved for use in Canada or many other countries such as Australia, New Zealand, and those in the EU. Why not? Are those nations' regulators, and the experts who advise them, right, and the United States wrong? And why has Canada resisted pressure to approve these drugs? There are two sides to the controversy.

No one denies that rBST can be a boon for dairy farmers. When cows are injected with this hormone every fourteen days, they increase their milk production by as much as 16 percent (in a few cases, even 40 percent increases have been recorded). With high feed costs and relatively low milk prices, why not make the extra profit? Besides, making cows more productive cuts greenhouse-gas emissions. This is good for the environment. Right?

Yes, in some ways it is great, but there are problems. Even the supporters reluctantly agree that it may have some very unpleasant health effects on the cattle—including mastitis (inflammation of the udders), lameness (due to hoof splitting), and infections at the hormone injection site. As I read it, Canada's resistance (as well as the position of such countries as Australia and New Zealand) seems to be mainly based on such effects on the poor cows.

But what about implications for us? These are less clear. Canada and other countries that are against the practice refer to "unanswered questions." True, we don't have a final answer. This is in spite of the reassurances by the manufacturer, the FDA, WHO, AMA, National Institutes of Health (NIH), ADA, and regulatory agencies in some thirty countries. Yes, Monsanto may be right in saying that rBST is one of the most researched animal products ever approved by the FDA. But investigative reports and lawsuits have argued that the company has tried to hide some of the most negative findings of those same studies. Also, as usual, we don't really know about any long-term negative effects—not months, but years away . . . and perhaps caused indirectly.

Two indirect problems *have* been flagged by critics of such rBST use. One is that the hormone-treated cows produce a little more of another compound—the insulin-like growth factor (IGF-1). Pasteurization does not destroy it, but some say that the digestive process would and others disagree. Although experts do not agree whether the amounts concerned are big enough, it has been suggested that increases of IGF-1 in milk could lead to early puberty in girls and increased risk of breast and colon cancer in adult women and men. I also found studies saying that a woman's chance of conceiving fraternal twins could be increased by IGF-1. Furthermore, studies have found that if males have high levels of IGF-1, their risk of developing prostate cancer can be raised four-fold. As a result, some doctors advise at-risk patients to use hormone-free dairy products, but such advice may come too late in life. However, other studies and experts have concluded that there is no proof of such negative effects on humans.

Now to the other possible human-health effect of Posilac use, which relates to the issue of bacteria in dairy. The fact that rBST cattle are having more cases of mastitis means that they will also be given more antibiotics. In turn, this could encourage other serious outcomes such as increased development of antibiotic-resistant bacteria (see following discussion of antibiotics).

Like many issues in food safety, the use of growth hormone for dairy cattle has resulted in a lot of contradictory and confusing opinions and arguments on both sides of the debate. We could get the definitive research findings any day. In the meantime, people at high risk or being treated for breast, prostate, or colon cancer may want to consume only organic, pasteurized milk and dairy products, or those labeled with some variation of "hormone-free," just in case further research *does* confirm these health risks.

A PITCHED BATTLE
OVER A MILK LABEL

Many American consumers have been worried about the use of hormones for a long time, particularly when the drugs are given to cattle that produce the milk their children drink. What they preferred was for the use of hormones to be banned. But if that was impossible, the second best choice was a label on milk cartons saying when hormones had been used, and when not.

All this seemed quite straightforward. But it wasn't. The way Monsanto, the industrial producer of the hormone at the time, and some dairy organizations saw it, if the milk label said that the milk was hormone-free, it implied that any milk that did contain hormones wasn't as good. Besides, they argued, all milk has *some* hormones in it, which is true. But it wasn't these normal levels of hormones that mothers were worried about. They were worried about the addition of new hormones, and an *unnatural* increase in the levels of the normal or "natural" ones.

To cut a long story short, the battle went on for about a year, with some states and some dairy producers supporting the industry position, and many other states and a few brave dairy producers (I live in fear of Monsanto) on the opposite side. In the end, Monsanto was unsuccessful in persuading the federal officials to crack down on labeling. Consumers got their way. But the industry did win part of the battle. By law, labels that say, "No hormones have been used" also have to include a disclaimer which essentially says, "No significant difference has been shown between milk derived from rBST treated or non-rBST treated cows."

Unfortunately, all this battle may have been for nothing. By the time hormone-free milk went onto the market, many people had lost interest. Few were willing to pay the higher price. Some already felt safe because they were purchasing organic milk. Then the recession hit. The bottom line: Sales did not meet expectations, and there was no discernible sales bump. At least that is what a study commissioned by Elanco—the new makers of Posilac—showed.

The Antibiotics Issue—Again

DAIRY COWS ARE often given antibiotics. Does this affect their milk, and should it concern us?

Dairy cattle, unlike beef cattle, are generally only given antibiotics and other **antimicrobial** drugs (such as sulfamethazine) to treat infections such as mastitis. Mastitis is the most common and costly infection found on dairy farms, although it is not the only one. It tends to be caused by *Staphylococcus* and *Streptococcus* bacteria (see also sidebar concerning hormone use). If this condition is left untreated, it is miserable for the poor cows. It also results in more bacteria in the milk they produce, which creates issues for dairy owners, and maybe, for us. Giving dairy cattle antibiotics helps to solve both these problems. A wide range of such antibiotics are given to cattle for mastitis and other cattle conditions (such as pneumonia, diarrhea, foot rot, uterine infections, pinkeye, and more). They include members of the penicillin, tetracycline, and other drug families. These kinds of antibiotics are also used in human medicine. This raises two issues we have met before: antibiotic residues and development of antibiotic-resistant bacteria.

It seems that if your concern is antibiotic residues in milk, you don't need to worry. Federal and state regulators in North America have established tolerance levels for all the approved antibiotics, and systems are in place to make sure that any milk that reaches the market is free from antibiotic residues. Routine tests for drug residues are performed on all milk entering dairy plants, and dairy farmers are aware of these. Even though it may seem like a waste, if antibiotics are given to sick dairy cattle, farmers have to discard the milk for several days as instructed on the label of the antibiotic to allow the residues to be eliminated from the cows' system. If dairy farmers let residue-laden milk get into the human milk supply, the chances are that they will be caught and fined. No one wants to fail the "cattle drug test." According to the National Dairy Council, in the United States, testing for animal drug residues (including antibiotics) has only come up positive in about one in a thousand tankers of milk, which is, of course, rejected for human use. But, as mentioned in connection with drug residues in meat (see page 146), we may be getting those antibiotic residues from our veal instead, because of this waste milk being given to young calves.

The issue of bacteria developing resistance to antibiotics has two answers. If milk cattle are indeed only given antibiotics occasionally for therapeutic purposes, and the instructions are correctly followed, this should not result in significant and lasting resistance developing among the target bacteria (or others affected by the drugs). However, if dairy cattle are being given regular small subtherapeutic doses (as reportedly some in North America are, but the frequency is not known), the situation changes. In this case, there is a greater chance of superbugs developing. The reasons are the same as when these practices are used with beef cattle, other food animals, or farmed fish: not all the bacteria will be wiped out by such low doses, and those tougher "survivor" bacteria will multiply and be more able to resist such drugs. And then, they could even swap genes with other bacteria and pass on this ability. These antibiotic-resistant bacteria could end up in milk if it is not pasteurized, and be a major risk for people who consume unpasteurized dairy. In addition, excreted antibiotic-resistant bacteria can also be **environmental contaminants**. From there, they may end up on vegetables and even fruit crops through contaminated irrigation water or runoff.

Again, it is raw milk drinkers and raw dairy eaters who are most at risk. But maybe even raw vegetable eaters, from the literal trickle-down effect.

POPs and Rocket Fuel in Our Milk?

I HAVE READ several studies and statistics that contend that fatty milk and dairy products contribute more to our body's POP levels than does any other food we eat, except perhaps fatty meat and fish. Research has found DDT metabolites in fatty cheeses and butter, dioxins in milk and other dairy, dieldrin in whole-milk yogurt, and PCBs in ice cream. These are just some examples. Some of these POPs are known to be carcinogenic. Within the human body, the highest levels of many of them are in body fat and breast milk, which has raised controversy about breast-feeding. Whether POPs and other toxic chemicals in our environment enter our milk and dairy products depends on whether they are in the dairy cow's feed and are able to pass the blood-milk barrier. The good news is that since the 1980s, levels of POPs, including dioxins, have been declining, both in the environment and in our body. That doesn't mean they are gone yet. Even very small doses can cause a variety of negative health effects, so it is best to keep our body levels as low as possible. The developing fetus is often most susceptible, arguing for the need for pregnant women to take special care.

In North America, levels of such toxic substances in food are monitored to protect our health, including in milk and milk products. However, some experts argue that the established "safe" levels are too high, particularly in the case of the more vulnerable fetus, as well as for toddlers who drink a lot of milk for their body weight. Older children and adults may also be exposed to these substances from not just dairy but several additional food sources as well, such as meat, fruits and vegetables, poultry, and fish.

As with our seafood, there may be greater reason to be concerned about the safety of our dairy imports, such as milk protein products. Some of these increasingly come from countries that have badly polluted environments and poor food safety practices and regulations. Contaminated imported ingredients in dairy cattle feed could also insert such hazards into our domestic dairy. A case that occurred in Germany could also be replicated here. In that instance, dairy products were heavily contaminated with dioxins. It was found that the dioxins originated in citrus pulp, imported from Brazil, that had been used in the cattle feed. Cases of dioxin contamination of cattle feed have also occurred in the United States, although there is little data on how this was reflected in dairy products. The research reviewed seems to argue that butter and cheese are our most risky dairy foods in terms of toxic POPs such as dioxins. But there is a great deal we still don't know about how much such toxic chemicals constitute a health risk in North America.

Of course, dioxins are not the only toxic chemical that might turn up in our dairy. There are others as well. Such as rocket fuel.

We don't want rocket fuel in our baby's formula, no matter how much new parenthood may be exhausting us. But it can happen. In fact, studies have found that children under ten years of age are most likely to have high perchlorate levels in their blood. It was concluded that this was probably because young children consumed more foods that were contaminated with this chemical from such sources as milk.

Perchlorate is a naturally occurring and man-made chemical that is a component of solid rocket fuel, fireworks, flares, and some fertilizers. We usually worry about perchlorate in public drinking water systems. But it can also be present in certain foods— including dairy. If present at sufficiently high levels, the functioning of the thyroid gland can be affected. It has been believed that perchlorate could be a particularly serious threat to the fetus and infants, affecting development of their central nervous system. However, some recent studies argue that such fears have been exaggerated.

A little-publicized study published in the March 2009 edition of the *Journal of Exposure Science and Environmental Epidemiology* reports that CDC scientists found fifteen brands of commercially available powdered infant formula to be contaminated with this toxic chemical. The data suggest that perchlorate-contaminated water used in making all the baby foods was one factor. But it turns out that the foods containing cows' milk ingredients were the *most* contaminated. This indicated that perchlorate was present in the milk as well.

The fact that milk and dairy products can be adding to our already too-high body burden of toxic chemicals is certainly bad news. One way we can limit some, like dioxins, is to consume low-fat or nonfat milk and dairy products and be very careful about which infant formulas we use.

Melamine Is Still There

MELAMINE ADULTERATION OF food hit the news in 2006–2007. Yes, it is an industrial chemical, but the case was so different from chemicals that enter accidentally that it deserves separate discussion.

Melamine is used in the manufacturing of plastics, flame retardants, and other such products. It is not approved for use in food. First there was the widespread melamine contamination of pet food in the United States. Then in fall 2008, we learned of melamine-contaminated infant formula in China, which sickened tens of thousands of children, led to the hospitalization of at least thirteen thousand, and resulted in several deaths. Melamine in combination with cyanuric acid (a mild acid, which can occur as an impurity of melamine) is worse than either alone. Together they form a deadly kidney-damaging partnership. We saw what happened to our beloved cats and dogs. We hate to even imagine what happened to those poor infants in China. These horrible incidents frightened us and left us feeling vulnerable to our globalized food supply.

Profit-motivated **food terrorism**, which is what this was, could happen so easily. All it took was some Chinese middlemen watering down the milk they collected from local farmers. They then added a dose of melamine to falsify the protein readings on tests, so that no one found out. Such melamine-contaminated milk was sold—apparently for years—to large companies that made products such as powdered milk. These companies then sold these to other companies both in China and overseas. The milk products of over twenty Chinese companies tested positive for melamine to a greater or lesser level. According to various press reports,

Chinese officials knew for months about the contaminated milk powder but took no action, no doubt because of the political and personal repercussions of reporting such things.

In a way, the melamine scandal was a wake-up call for many countries. How can we check for every possible toxic chemical in the food that crosses our borders? We are now importing large amounts of milk-derived products from China, particularly casein, caseinates and derivatives, and other milk proteins, as well as some yogurt, butter, and processed cheese. These melamine incidents resulted in U.S. and Canadian action to keep potentially contaminated milk products and foods out. Those suspect foods that had already been imported were quickly checked for any melamine presence. We found to our dismay that testing for melamine had to go beyond any foods imported from China itself. Contaminated products could also reach us indirectly from other countries using tainted imported ingredients from China and then exporting the finished foods to us. A globalized food supply makes safety a much more complicated issue.

In fact, melamine did turn up in high levels in certain foods already on the market in the United States and Canada, many of them unfortunately targeted to children. The first recalls involved many products that children love: candies, milk drinks, and cookies with appealing animal names and pictures on labels (cats, rabbits, koalas), eaten primarily by the Chinese community. Soon other products such as instant coffee and tea blends turned up positive as well. My spot checks during the recalls showed that at least some small markets were still selling these recalled items weeks after the FDA had sent out the recalls.

But then we had even more news. The FDA and USDA testing for melamine revealed that low levels of melamine and cyanuric acid can be present in a whole range of our foods. In fact, it *can* get in accidentally: Melamine is present in many food packaging materials, some sprays used to clean processing equipment, and some insecticides sprayed on animals and crops. The FDA stated that such low levels are "deemed safe" and do not pose a health risk. New FDA guidelines limited melamine levels to below 2.5 parts per million (ppm) in food and to 1 ppm in infant food.

But there is a great deal we still don't know. My reading of the expert reviews of the FDA decision and of the toxicology studies performed (see appendix 4) confirmed what I suspected. Studies have not looked sufficiently at risks over a long period of time (after all, we just recently discovered it was an issue in food), have not taken into account how risks could be compounded by melamine from several food sources, or examined the greater risk posed when melamine combines with other substances that may increase toxicity. Nor have standards adequately considered the greater vulnerability of toddlers and young children, pregnant and lactating women, the elderly, and people with chronic diseases whose kidneys and other body organs are underdeveloped or not functioning like those of healthy adults. In other words, this issue is still far from resolved. Even the FDA acknowledges that more studies are needed.

In the meantime, what can we do? Melamine and similar contaminants are impossible to avoid in almost any food that could pick it up during processing or from its packaging. When the melamine scandal was at its height, people asked me what they could do. All I could suggest was what I do myself: Eat as few processed foods as you can—and read the labels.

Read Those Labels

IT USED TO be that milk was just labeled "milk" or "pasteurized milk." These days, you could spend half your shopping time reading the labels on milk, cheese, yogurt, butter, and other dairy products. Some of these are useful from a safety perspective.

Pasteurized

When a dairy product is labeled "pasteurized," it means that it has been heated to a certain specified temperature for a specified period of time to kill pathogenic (disease-causing) organisms without harming the flavor or quality of the food. Pasteurization of milk and other dairy has to use one of the several approved methods (see page 179). Although pasteurization may not kill every single bacterium or inactivate every possible toxin, the "pasteurized" label is usually interpreted as meaning that the milk or other dairy product is most likely to be safe.

Organic

As with other foods, *certified organic* means that the milk or milk product adheres to the standards of the USDA's National Organics Program. Organic milk comes from cows that have not been given antibiotics or artificial hormones, and no pesticides, herbicides, or chemical fertilizers have been used on their grazing land or feed. Feed has to be grown on land that has met these organic conditions for at least three years. Certifying agents review farmer applications for organic dairy certification, and inspectors carry out on-site inspections. Farm records have to be kept to document that the producers are keeping to the organic requirements. Such requirements increase costs to the farmer, particularly during the transition period, and these are passed on to the consumer.

Hormone-free

Milk labeled "hormone-free" or "free of artificial growth hormones" or something similar comes from dairies that have agreed not to give the cows hormones of any kind. This label came after a long battle about the issue, and in response to strong consumer demand, and has to be followed by a disclaimer (see page 194). Contrary to the requirements for an organic label, apparently U.S. "hormone-free" dairy farms are not inspected. In most cases, those farmers sign a legally binding affidavit instead.

. . .

Probiotic

When yogurt is labeled "probiotic," it means that it contains "friendly" bacteria such as those normally found in the intestinal tract, which aid digestion. They include such bacteria as *Bifidobacterium bifidus*, *Lactobacillus acidophilus*, *L. bulgaricus*, *L. casei*, and *Streptococcus thermophilus*.

To help consumers distinguish between which was which, the National Yogurt Association (a nonprofit U.S. trade association) developed the "Live and Active Cultures" seal. For manufacturers to carry the seal, refrigerated yogurt products must contain at least a hundred million bacteria cultures per gram at the time of manufacture, and frozen yogurt products must contain ten million cultures per gram at the time of manufacture. This program is voluntary, which means that some manufacturers of live-culture yogurt may simply prefer not to use the seal.

Certified

Milk labeled "certified" can be either pasteurized or raw, but has to be produced according to the laws and sanitation regulations of the American Association of Medical Milk Commissions, Inc. These regulations are fairly strict and are outlined in a special manual, which is revised on a regular basis. Dairy farmers who want this certification have to undergo inspections of their farm and equipment to determine it is sanitary, examinations of cows by veterinarians, and even health inspections of their employees. The demand for certified milk remains low and is not growing at the pace of demand for organic milk, but it should certainly be safer than milk that is not certified.

USDA Grades

The USDA grade shield on a cheese means that the cheese has been produced in a USDA-approved plant, under sanitary conditions, and has been inspected and graded by a government grader according to USDA Marketing Service guidelines. Not all types of cheese are eligible. You are most likely to find the shield on a Monterey Jack, Cheddar, Colby, or Swiss cheese. The shield should offer a greater assurance of safety as well as quality on such cheeses.

But What About . . . ?

How can I keep milk fresh?

When buying milk, always choose the milk container with the "best before" date furthest into the future, so that it is freshest. Once home, it should be put immediately into the refrigerator— on the refrigerator shelves, not the doors, which are usually not cold enough. To avoid milk's getting "off" flavors and smells, leave it in its original container and keep the containers closed and away from other strong-smelling foods. Once you open a can of milk or an aseptic UHT (ultra-high temperature) milk product, it must be refrigerated, too. Before it is opened, UHT milk can be kept for up to four months, and for two months in the fridge after it is opened. Powdered milk can be stored unopened for up to a year.

Is milk safe after the sell-by date?

Yes, milk can be kept quite a while beyond the sell-by date if it has been kept on a shelf in the refrigerator and didn't get too warm on the way home from the store (see following chart for specifics). It is easy to tell when milk is spoiled by the unpleasant smell (like baby's vomit). This means that spoilage bacteria are at work—not necessarily ones that make you ill. But who wants to drink milk that smells like that? Yogurt may be kept even a bit longer after the sell-by date, although there may be a slight change in its texture over time.

Can milk be safely frozen?

Yes, milk can be frozen for about three weeks. However, there will be minor nutrient loss, and the texture may change slightly, too, less so with skim milk or 2% milk than with whole milk.

Should I remove cheese from its original wrapping after I open it?

Refrigerate all cheeses between 35° and 40°F in their original wrapping until you are ready to eat them. Like milk, cheeses can pick up "off" flavors from other foods, so it is best to keep them in the refrigerator drawer, or away from smelly foods. Once you take the cheese out of the packaging you bought it in, wrap it tightly with new plastic wrap, making sure there are no air pockets. If you are concerned about DEHA leaching out of the plastic wrap into the cheese, use a brand that does not have it (check the results of Consumers Union testing).

How long can I keep cheese after I buy it?

That depends on the type of cheese, and, of course, what condition it is in when you buy it. The general opinion seems to be that in the refrigerator you can keep hard cheese for two to four weeks, soft cheese (such as ricotta, cottage cheese, Brie, and Camembert) for only five to seven days, Parmesan or Romano cheese for as long as two to three months, and processed cheese products for three to four weeks (see also the following chart). If you have had that Brie or Camembert cheese sitting on the platter in a warm room for more than four hours while you waited for your guests to eat it, throw it out or put it in the dog dish. But you may want to put the dog outside afterward in case it throws it up.

Is organic milk safer than regular milk?

The National Dairy Council says organic milk is the same as nonorganic milk in terms of both nutrition value and safety. Both the National Dairy Council and state bodies such as the

California Dairy Council claim that established government standards, which include testing milk for antibiotic and pesticide residue, ensure that conventional milk is just as safe as organic milk. Of course, there are plenty of people who disagree with that position. In the end, it boils down to whom you believe.

Smart Ways to Reduce Your Risks

As USUAL, YOU need to pay most attention to safety risks in dairy products if you are in one of the high-risk groups: pregnant women or women considering pregnancy, children under five years of age, the elderly, those infected with HIV, people with cancer or under treatment, and anyone else who has a weakened immune system (such as persons with organ transplants and with certain chronic diseases). Luckily, being a smart dairy consumer is not very complicated. The most important rule is a simple one: Only drink milk or eat dairy products that are pasteurized. That will at least protect you from most of the bacteria in milk. If you want to be supersafe, you may want to drink organic pasteurized milk or follow that "know your cow" rule. Apart from that, just make smart dairy decisions.

Buy milk and dairy products carefully. Read the label on dairy and always make sure the word *pasteurized* appears somewhere on it. When shopping at places such as farmers' markets, where products may not always be fully labeled, be sure to ask. If you want to avoid added hormones, then buy organic or "hormone-free" dairy. If you want to reduce not just your access to extra hormones but to antibiotic-resistant bacteria, buying organic dairy may also help. The cows producing such milk are likely to have received fewer antibiotics, if any, and not be given rBST. It can also be argued that organic dairy is likely to contain lower levels of agricultural chemicals, but there is no guarantee that it will be free of the industrial ones.

Drink and eat pasteurized dairy. Never drink raw milk or eat any dairy product—cheeses, or anything else—that has been made from raw milk. Only eat aged raw milk cheeses if you are very healthy.

Stick to low- or nonfat dairy. Among other things, this will help you lower your intake of POPs and other toxic chemicals from dairy foods. The USDA advice for all adults and children over the age of two is to keep to low-fat dairy. (Children under two years of age need milk with a higher fat content.)

Consider the yogurt alternative. A few studies have found that yogurt eaters end up with less heavy metals in their body, and that fermentation may help to degrade certain chemical toxins as well. These claims are not proven. But who knows?

Store correctly. Dairy requires storage in the refrigerator. Store milk on the shelves of your refrigerator. Store cheese at 35° to 45°F in the refrigerator. Throw out any dairy that smells odd or is moldy, except in the case of hard cheese (when you can carefully trim off the mold with a half- to one-inch margin around it). Remember—the roots of the mold can penetrate farther than you can see. After any trimming, use fresh wrap for the cheese and throw out the removed part carefully. Make sure you do not keep dairy beyond the recommended times (see chart).

• • •

SAFE DAIRY STORAGE

Type of Dairy	How to Store	How Long to Store in Refrigerator (35°–40°F) for Best Quality and Safety
Pasteurized fresh milk	Refrigerate in original container. Keep container closed.	1–5 days from sell-by date
Butter	Refrigerate in original wrapper or covered butter dish.	Up to 1 month
Sweet cream	Refrigerate in original closed container.	1–4 days from sell-by date
Yogurt	Refrigerate covered.	7–10 days
Sour cream, buttermilk	Refrigerate in original container. Keep container closed.	2 weeks
Dairy desserts (such as custards, milk puddings)	Cool cooked dishes quickly and refrigerate, covered, within 2 hours. Refrigerate cold-prepared dishes immediately, covered, after preparation.	5–6 days
Natural hard and semihard cheese (such as brick, Cheddar, Swiss, Parmesan) and processed cheese	Refrigerate in original wrapper. Once opened, either overwrap or rewrap tightly with plastic wrap or place in a closed plastic bag, to prevent drying.	Up to 1 month
Soft cheese (such as Camembert, Brie, cottage, cream, Limburger)	Refrigerate in original wrap or container, tightly covered, as above.	1 week
Cheese spreads	Refrigerate, tightly covered.	1 month
Canned milk (opened)	Refrigerate, tightly covered.	1 week
Whipped topping	Refrigerate, tightly covered.	In aerosol can: 3 months Prepared from mix: 3 days Bought frozen: 2 weeks (once thawed)

Always pay attention to contamination risks in your own kitchen. The case of dairy is no different from any other food. Cross-contamination is always a risk. Watch that cheese sitting next to the pâté or sliced roast beef on the tray!

Eat out with care. In the case of dairy foods, be careful with such dairy as cheeses at larger receptions and in restaurants. If you think they have been sitting out too long at a warm temperature, just pass. Eat the olives instead.

Take special care if you are in a high-risk group. Some doctors and practitioners of alternative medicine suggest that dairy products should be avoided completely by people with high IGF-1 levels and those who are at risk for breast or prostate cancer. Not everyone agrees. But if you are in such a group—and dairy is not too hard to give up—you may want to consider this advice (and get your calcium from other sources).

8

Eggs

The year 2010 may go down in U.S. food-safety history as "the year of the bad egg." There was a multistate recall of some half a billion shell eggs, at least 1,500 associated *Salmonella*-caused illnesses, newspapers loaded with articles about the recall, and confused consumers staring at empty store shelves. That was the year when many Americans realized for the first time that their perfect-looking, spotlessly clean eggs may not be as perfect as they appear. In fact, they can be downright dangerous. And it is not just those factory-farm eggs. Organic eggs, free-range eggs, omega-3 eggs, and all those other types of eggs and egg products are not risk-free, either.

Up until the 2010 outbreak, it appeared that risks in eggs had been decreased, although not been completely eliminated. In the United States, you could assume that about one out of every twenty thousand eggs might give you a case of food poisoning—more or less averaging one bad egg in a lifetime. After 2010 those odds may well have changed, particularly if you eat a lot of eggs. Your odds are also worse if you eat eggs in an institutional setting, such a school or nursing home, or consume them often in restaurant meals.

What We Eat

THE AMERICAN EGG Board will tell you that the "incredible edible egg" has amazing nutritional value. One egg has as many as thirteen essential nutrients, including high-quality protein, zinc, iron, choline, and folate, all for a low 75 calories. Eggs are good for our brain, our eyes, our energy, and much more. They are also relatively cheap. But holding egg consumption back is our fear of cholesterol and perhaps also our concern about how all those hard-working laying hens are being treated.

According to the egg industry statistics, the annual per-person egg consumption in the United States in 2008 was around 250 eggs. In Canada, the number of eggs eaten per person is somewhere between 144 and 181 (estimates vary)—down from around 276 in 1960. People in countries such as Mexico, China, and Japan eat many more eggs each year than we do.

Of the billions of eggs eaten each year by North Americans, roughly about two thirds are eaten as "shell eggs" and the other third as "egg products."

Shell Eggs

Shell eggs—those whole eggs we buy in the cartons—can spoil, just like fruit, meat, fish and other fresh food products. They can be contaminated right in the shell even before they show any visible signs. Normally, shell eggs on the market are unpasteurized. However, pasteurized shell eggs are now being sold in some stores. These are easy to recognize: The FDA requires that each egg be marked to indicate that it has been pasteurized, or that the carton be shrink-wrapped or otherwise packaged in some way that allows the buyer to tell whether it has been opened (which might jeopardize the purity of the pasteurized eggs).

Egg Products

Egg products are eggs removed from their shells, and can be liquid, frozen, or dried whole eggs, whites, yolks, or blends of egg and other ingredients. "Egg substitutes" can be liquid or frozen, and only contain the egg white. Egg products and egg substitutes are pasteurized. They are therefore safer from microbe contaminants—including that nasty *Salmonella* bacteria—than are unpasteurized shell eggs.

Egg products are used much more extensively by restaurants and institutional kitchens now than they were a decade ago. They are also gaining popularity with consumers, particularly in the form of liquid refrigerated eggs. After all, why waste time cracking messy eggs when you can just pour from a carton? Convenience is in. Egg products are probably the only instance in our food supply where convenience means more safety, rather than less.

Specialty Egg Products

Increasingly popular specialty egg products go a step further, in terms of convenience. But often they are a step *down*, in terms of safety. They include prepared items that salad bars like, such as chopped hard-cooked eggs. They also include those egg products home cooks find convenient, the kind that just pop into the microwave or pot, or can be eaten without cooking, such as frozen quiche mixes, frozen scrambled eggs in a boilable pouch, freeze-dried scrambled eggs (which are handy for camping), omelets, and egg patties, and freeze-dried precooked scrambled eggs.

. . .

Who Keeps It Safe?

GOVERNMENT AND THE egg industry try to make sure that our eggs and egg products remain uncontaminated every step of the way from that long-suffering hen to our plate: during production, processing, and packing; transportation; retail; and consumption. Much of the safety focus is on the inspection, refrigeration, and labeling of eggs and egg products. For a long time, the major goal has been to avoid contamination of eggs by *Salmonella* bacteria.

In Canada, CFIA inspectors monitor egg operations and conduct testing to make sure that safety regulations and product standards are being kept to. The Canadian Egg Marketing Agency has developed a code for farm management that helps egg producers watch out for safety risks and apply good safety standards.

For some reason that escapes me, in the United States, the FDA and USDA/FSIS (plus some other agencies as well) share authority for egg safety. In general terms, the FDA is the key agency for production and processing of *fresh* eggs (eggs in their shells), and the USDA/ FSIS takes the lead in ensuring safety of liquid, frozen, and dried egg products, as well as any imported eggs destined for those products. In practice, the latter agency has some involvement with shell eggs as well.

As usual, the states play a key role in actual hands-on inspection activities. They may have their own additional laws governing eggs, consistent with the federal laws and standards. Under FDA and USDA/FSIS guidance, state-level activities mainly focus on how eggs are packed and shipped within state borders and how they are handled by stores and the food-service industry.

One Bad *Salmonella* Egg Too Many

THE BIGGEST SAFETY risk in eggs is the bacterium *Salmonella enteritidis* (SE)—the one that was also involved in the huge 2010 outbreak and recall. Even prior to 2010, the FDA estimates that, on average, 142,000 Americans became ill each year from consuming *Salmonella*-contaminated "bad" eggs. Repeated efforts over the years have failed to wipe SE out completely. To make this issue more frightening, many *Salmonella* spp. bacteria are now developing antibiotic resistance. The good news is that if this bacterium is present in our eggs, usually proper cooking or pasteurization will put it out of action. The problem is that many people still eat undercooked eggs or dishes made with undercooked eggs. Some studies in America have found that about a third of the time that people eat eggs, they ate undercooked eggs. Research in Canada has found that the elderly—who are also the most likely to get seriously ill from *Salmonella* infections—tend to become ill from undercooked eggs most often (but there could be several reasons for this, including higher egg consumption in general).

Improvements *have* been made to reduce this egg-related risk in our food. In the United States, many of these came after the huge *Salmonella* epidemic in the 1980s, which spread to 45 percent of America's egg-laying flocks. Outbreaks were particularly bad in certain parts of the country. Reduction of *Salmonella* bacteria in eggs was achieved on poultry farms (laying hens who test positive for SE tend to lay contaminated eggs) and during egg transport (correct refrigeration is important to keep SE numbers down). Efforts were also made to educate consumers and the food-service industry. As a result, SE incidents in the United States were cut to about half. But, as shown by the 2010 outbreak, still more effort is needed to improve egg safety, particularly at the farm level. On July 9, 2010, the new federal rule to lower the risk of *Salmonella*-tainted eggs (entitled "Prevention of Salmonella Enteritidis in Shell Eggs During Production, Storage, and Transportation") went into effect. Full compliance by all larger egg producers (with three thousand or more laying hens—about 99 percent of total) and by egg transporters was targeted for July 2012. Mainly, the new regulations focus on strengthening and systematizing existing *Salmonella*-prevention measures at the farm level and enforcing careful refrigeration of eggs during storage and transport. Implementation of the procedures is expected to reduce U.S. egg-associated instances of salmonellosis by nearly 60 percent—with $1.4 billion in public health savings.

Presently, *Salmonella* outbreaks in our eggs still occur every year. Usually they are relatively small and localized. Occasionally, they are almost nationwide, as in 2010, and involve huge producers. No type of egg is really safe from SE, whether it be organic, natural, "vegetarian," or any other kind (see sidebar). In March 2009, for instance, due to *Salmonella*, there was a recall of brown organic eggs produced in Ripon, California, by a safety-conscious private poultry farm. It had been operating for more than fifty years and supplied eggs to such major retail outlets as Costco, Safeway, and Pac "N" Save stores.

HOW *SALMONELLA* BACTERIA ENTER THE EGG

Yes, it is true—those perfect eggs, which look so clean and innocent, can actually be contaminated with dangerous bacteria. And not just on the outside. Contrary to what most of us have always believed, shell eggs may have *Salmonella* bacteria on the inside even when the shell is clean and unbroken. Bacteria usually enter eggs at the farm level. They can be present in the oviduct of laying chickens and enter the eggs before the shell forms around it. The chickens themselves can look perfectly healthy.

Some research studies argue that the industry profit-motivated practice of forced molting laying hens (essentially by starving them to manipulate egg laying by the hens—also an animal-rights issue) encourages such bacteria to increase in numbers and virulence. This would make sense in terms of the generally opportunistic behavior of bacteria—attacking when their victim is weaker. Contamination can also take place after the egg has been laid, with bacteria originating in floor litter and fecal material. Insects, rodents, and the hens, themselves, help to spread it. The crowded conditions of factory farming are a major factor. The longer the eggs stay in the laying house after being laid, the more chance there is of bacteria getting in.

The egg *does* have many built-in barriers, including the shell and the membrane beneath it. But bacteria are remarkably persistent. It seems that the *Salmonella* bacteria first enter the white of the egg, where they multiply slowly. As the egg ages and barriers break down, they are able to enter the nutrient-rich yolk. If the temperature is attractive, they increase their numbers rapidly. One bacterium can become over a million bacteria within hours. Not a pleasant thought.

Although it is the most common, SE is not the only type of microorganism that can crop up in our eggs. However, only a small percentage—around 3 percent—of dangerous egg contamination is caused by other bacteria such as *Staphylococcus aureus* or by viruses such as norovirus. Spoilage bacteria can also get in, including *Pseudomonas* (which can give eggs an odd fruity smell and a blue-green coloring), and *Flavobacteria*. These bacteria are unlikely to make us ill.

Even pasteurized egg products—both liquid and dried—can become contaminated, although much more rarely. In such cases, the culprit is usually not SE, but the dangerous *Listeria* bacteria (see page 186). It is believed that they do not enter at the farm level, but originate instead from *Listeria*-carrying people who work in egg-processing plants. Some scientists contend that if the *Listeria* bacteria are present in large enough numbers in eggs *before* they are pasteurized, the presently used pasteurization temperatures may not be high enough to kill them all. *Listeria* can even increase in numbers in refrigerated egg products and survive in frozen ones.

Of course, *Salmonella, Listeria,* and any of a number of other bacteria can also enter a cracked-open shell egg or unpackaged egg product if put into contact with another contaminated food. Contamination can happen, for instance, when an egg product is mixed with another item in a restaurant and left sitting for a while (as in a prepared omelet mix).

To avoid picking up a bacterium from your eggs, you need to remember that some types of whole-egg dishes are riskier than others. *Salmonella* illnesses have often been linked to scrambled eggs, eggs Benedict, fried eggs, and omelets—served in restaurants, institutions, and private homes. Other lightly cooked or uncooked dishes that use raw egg as an ingredient are also common causes of illness. Most of these incidents occur on a small scale—among members of a family or diners at a single restaurant. Take a friend of mine, who had been eating eggs at the same San Francisco restaurant for years, with no problems. The chef changed, and one day her poached egg was softer than usual. She was late for work, so she didn't send the dish back—only to severely regret it a few hours later. I know another person who came down with severe salmonellosis one day after eating egg drop soup at a local Chinese restaurant from which she had been ordering it for nearly a decade without becoming ill. (She has not gone back there since.)

These days, the commercially prepared versions of the dishes in the sidebar, and those served at restaurants, are usually made with pasteurized egg products. They are therefore safer—unless contaminated later. Some of the more recent outbreaks involving such foods have occurred at upper-end restaurants that still use whole eggs.

KNOW YOUR RISKY EGG DISHES

◇ **Breakfast dishes:** French toast, pancakes, soft-boiled and sunny-side up eggs
◇ **Ready-to-eat foods:** deli egg salads, sandwiches
◇ **Main dishes:** crab cakes; casseroles; eggs Benedict; omelets; pasta carbonara, as well as lasagne, ravioli, and other stuffed pasta dishes containing eggs; egg drop soup; stir-fries (including fried rice) to which eggs are added during the last moments of cooking
◇ **Sauces and dressings:** béarnaise sauce, Caesar salad dressing, freshly made mayonnaise, hollandaise sauce
◇ **Desserts:** cakes or pies with chiffon or custard fillings or

> meringue toppings; egg-containing creams, custard, floating islands, mousse, soufflés, and tiramisu; home-made ice cream and gelato; unbaked dessert batters/doughs that contain eggs (see sidebar, page 246)
>
> ◇ **Drinks:** eggnog, "health food" milkshakes that contain egg, "prairie oyster" hangover concoctions that contain raw egg

Even if you encounter a *Salmonella*-contaminated egg just once in your life, that could be once too many, particularly if you eat it while your natural defenses are down, or when you need to be at your best. If your "bad egg" turn comes up, and you unknowingly pool it with others to make undercooked scrambled egg for your whole family, then you share the risk. But remember—as in the case of meat—if you cook that egg well, you are unlikely to become ill. Both pasteurized liquid egg and pasteurized whole eggs are normally attractive options for high-risk people such as pregnant women, those with weakened immune systems, older adults, and infants and young children.

Forget About Bird Flu

AVIAN INFLUENZA IS a frightening disease that has crossed the species barrier from birds to humans. It is discussed in more detail in chapter 6. Here, it is only mentioning in passing because of consumer concerns. Could the virus that causes avian influenza also get into our eggs?

True, where birds have the virus, it may also be present in the eggs they lay—*if* they lay any. In such cases it can be both on the outside shell and in the white and yolk of the egg. However, the good news is that hens stop laying eggs soon after they are infected. The other good news is that, in the United States and Canada, bird flu–infected eggs would be eliminated during the washing and grading processes because they are usually weak and misshapen (although other factors can also cause such eggs). The third piece of good news is that if there were a suspected outbreak of avian influenza among laying hens, regulators would immediately stop any poultry or eggs from reaching the market, even before test results are in. Finally, in the very remote case that this virus did get into eggs, it would be inactivated by proper pasteurization or cooking (the USDA laboratories checked this just to make sure). In sum, bird flu in your eggs should not be at the top of your worry list for now—particularly if you stick to well-cooked eggs.

Is Antibiotic Use an Issue?

WHEN LAYING HENS become ill with diseases such as fowl pox, Newcastle disease, and bronchitis, they are often given antibiotics. Any such use of any antibiotics is strictly regulated by the FDA and the USDA. As with meat animals, and with dairy cattle, a withdrawal period following antibiotic use is also required to cleanse the bird's system.

In theory, laying hens are not given any subtherapeutic antibiotics—that is, low doses in their feed simply to keep them healthy and make sure they continue laying. But there are reports all over the place that this is being done anyway. If this is true, then it could be playing a role in the developing resistance of SE bacteria to antibiotics, as such practices could be doing in the case of meat-type poultry production (see page 140). It is difficult to find reliable data on this issue.

Regulators and the egg industry say that eggs are safe from any antibiotic residue, because of two reasons: the withdrawal period imposed, and because laying hens usually do not produce many eggs anyway while they are ill. But there are reports suggesting that low levels of such drug residues persist longer than is commonly assumed and do, in fact, turn up both in the white and yolk of the egg. According to some estimates, as many as 10 percent of eggs on the U.S. market contain drug residues, including of some drugs that are being used to control intestinal parasites in poultry, which have not been evaluated for human safety. However, several of the research studies reviewed have come up with only around 3 percent, and the levels have been low. Compared to all the other risks in our food, drug residues in eggs appear to be a relatively minor issue. But if you are worried, there is the organic alternative, or eggs labeled "no antibiotics used."

Read Those Labels

EGG CARTONS NOW tend to have a wide variety of labels. The below discussion of labels applies to the United States. There are close parallels with Canada.

Inspection Marks

The USDA grade mark on shell egg cartons means the plant that processed the eggs is following the USDA's sanitation and good manufacturing processes. Officially inspected egg products also have the USDA inspection mark.

Egg Grading

As with other food products, such as meat, grading of eggs is voluntary. About 40 percent of U.S. eggs are graded from A or AA for their external appearance (clean, unbroken shells), weight, and interior quality (see figure 8). This grading means little, if anything, in terms of safety.

Figure 8

Dating on Egg Cartons

Dating of eggs is important in terms of safety. Egg cartons with the USDA grade shield on them are required to have a *pack date* (the day that the eggs were washed, graded, and placed in the carton).

The number is a modified use of the Julian date, namely a three-digit code that refers to the consecutive days of the year (January 20 would be 020, March 1 would be 063 and so on, to December 31 being 365). Although not required by federal law, state laws may require egg cartons to have a sell-by or expiration date. If there is a sell-by date on a carton with a USDA grade shield, then it cannot exceed the packing date by more than 45 days. It may be less if the producer or a supermarket prefers it that way.

Pasteurized

Pasteurized eggs are heated to a temperature that is high enough to kill most bacteria, including ones inside the egg, but not high enough to coagulate the eggs. These eggs are safer for use by people with a weakened immune system and those who prefer undercooked egg dishes (such as soft omelets or sunny-side up fried eggs) and for certain dishes that would leave the egg ingredient undercooked.

Cage-Free

Stores commonly carry labels on eggs saying they are "cage-free." This label basically means that up to seven hens are not locked up together in small battery cages, unable to flap a wing. They may instead spend their days crowded into a shed, one on top of another, struggling for space. However, if it makes you feel better, the Humane Society has endorsed this practice, as have some religious leaders. True, it is probably better than the usual egg factory farm—but marginally. I find it difficult to look at hens living under those conditions, remembering the happy hens I kept on the farm—and later, in our backyard. But hen welfare and egg safety are not necessarily connected. The research evidence is contradictory on whether cages or hen-laying houses are better in terms of hen hygiene (and therefore less likely to promote *Salmonella* contamination). Studies can be found to support either argument.

Free-Range

The USDA defines free-range as a step beyond "cage-free," in that these hens have at least limited access to the outdoors. But how exactly we define "the outdoors" is open to interpretation, especially in the case of laying hens. There is a big loophole in the law, which says that such access must be continuous "unless there is a health risk present." "Risk" is open to interpretation. It can mean anything: the weather is too cold; there may be a rat outside; or a wind may be blowing. Reports reveal that in practice some poultry farmers interpret *cage-free* and *free-range* as being the same thing. In other words, the supposedly free-range hens may never see the light of day, let alone a field of green grass and dandelions. They spend their lives in "indoor floor operations." (The European conditions for free-range eggs, by the way, are more specific and humane). Whether the eggs of so-called free-range hens are *safer* than those of caged ones is debatable, although you will certainly find claims that they are.

Hormone-Free or Antibiotic-Free

In the USDA's opinion these egg-carton labels are meaningless. In theory, all U.S. eggs are hormone-free (federal law prohibits use of hormones or steroids in poultry production) and antibiotic-free (any antibiotic residues would have been eliminated). However, if you don't quite trust that antibiotic residue elimination claim, you may want to buy them.

Organic

Eggs that are labeled organic and have the USDA organic seal on the carton were produced following the USDA National Organic Program standards (see page 78). The feed of hens producing organic eggs must be free of chemicals, such as pesticides, and meat products. Nor can they be given antibiotics, except in the case of an outbreak of disease. Usually their living conditions are also more humane.

Natural

Shell eggs are another instance of marketing-oriented use of the "natural" label. The USDA basically defines *natural* rather loosely, but makes it clear that it has nothing to do with the way a product is produced. To be labeled "natural," an item simply has to contain no artificial ingredients and be, at most, minimally processed. That certainly applies to all shell eggs, as they are only cleaned and graded, and have no ingredients added. Therefore *all* shell eggs are natural.

Vegetarian

Vegetarian eggs are produced by hens that are fed only a vegetarian diet—one with no meat or egg products included, presumably not even a bug. Hens are normally kept in cages. The eggs are also more expensive. The label has no safety significance.

Omega-3

The label "omega-3 enhanced" means that the laying hens have been given a special diet heavy in products that are rich in omega-3 fatty acids, such as canola (rapeseed), linseed, and flaxseed. As a result, these eggs contain higher than normal levels of wonderful omega-3. However, the hens may not have lived such wonderful lives, spending their days in small battery cages. This label has no importance in terms of safety, but you may prefer omega-3 eggs for nutritional reasons.

Safe Handling Instructions

In case you have ever wondered about the following, this label has to be there by federal law on all raw, unpasteurized shell eggs:

"SAFE HANDLING INSTRUCTIONS: To prevent illness from bacteria: Keep eggs refrigerated, cook eggs until yolks are firm, and cook foods containing eggs thoroughly." Have you ever read it? It's supposed to make us do our part.

But What About . . . ?

Can I tell by looking at an egg if it is fresh?

You can't tell if an egg is fresh by looking at it in the shell. However, if you are worried about the freshness of an egg, gently float it in a bowl of water. A fresh egg should sink. If it floats, it is likely to be getting old. In that case, crack it open in a separate dish and smell it. If it has an "off" odor, discard. Once you have cracked open a raw egg, you will have many more clues, besides odor. Contrary to what many people believe, if the egg white is cloudy or a boiled egg is hard to peel, this usually suggests freshness. If the egg white is clear, it is likely that the egg is beginning to age. (The air cell in the egg becomes larger). The appearance of the yolk is also a clue to freshness. When a fresh egg is being fried or poached, its yolk tends to hold its shape (be rounded). As an egg ages, the yolk becomes flatter and larger, and the white also spreads out more, but that does not necessarily mean it is unsafe. Fresh eggs also have clearly visible strands of egg white called "chalaza," which anchor the yolk in place, and it is perfectly safe to eat this. (The only time you need to take the chalaza out is if you are making stirred custard.) If an egg feels slimy, smells strange, or has spots on it, throw it out. In North America, commercially produced eggs usually arrive at stores a few days after they are laid, so unless the store has a slow turnover, they should be fresh when you buy them.

How long should eggs be cooked to be safe?

To make sure that the egg is safe to eat, it should be cooked until the yolk is firm—not runny. The consensus seems to be that eggs should be boiled about seven minutes, but some of us have found that it takes at least eight to nine minutes, with today's larger eggs. If poached, you should estimate about five minutes; and for fried, two to three minutes on each side. Scrambled eggs and omelets should be cooked until firm, leaving no runny areas. I always find this a challenge as I love to make interesting omelets but hate overcooked ones. This makes it a matter of temperature control and very precise timing. Some data show that many egg-borne illnesses come from underdone fried eggs (such as sunny-side up), so particularly watch those. And notice that there are *no* acceptable times for soft-boiled eggs.

Why are the eggs we buy so clean looking?

The eggs we buy in stores are thoroughly washed. Washing of eggs is also an important safety step. If you have ever worked on a poultry farm, as I have, you know what eggs look like when they are first laid. *Soiled* is a polite way of putting it. For safety reasons, government regulations call for those nasty-looking eggs to be carefully washed with special detergent and sanitized to remove dirt and fecal matter. Following this, the hen's original protective shell coating is replaced by a thin spray coating of natural mineral oil. Afterward, the egg looks much more attractive and more edible than when it first came out. However, all this may not be enough to keep bacteria out, and it certainly does not get rid of germs if they are already safely hiding inside.

Does the shell color have anything to do with egg quality or safety?

Chicken eggs can be white or brown or some shade in between. This has nothing to do with egg quality, nutritional value, flavor, safety, or freshness. If you think a brown egg tastes better, it probably just means that you are a New Englander or that you want to believe you are getting your money's worth since you paid more for them. The color of the shell is simply determined by the breed of the laying hen. If the hen has white feathers and white earlobes, the eggs turn out white. If it has red feathers and red earlobes (as in the case of the Rhode Island Red, Plymouth Rock, and New Hampshire hens), the eggs produced are brown. I still prefer my eggs brown, which goes to show how illogical one can be.

What do the different color pigmentations inside eggs mean?

The color of the yolk is simply a matter of the hen's diet. It does not mean anything in terms of egg quality, nutritional value, safety, or freshness. You will find claims that genuine free-range eggs have a more orange yolk and are of higher nutritional value, which is not true.

A very yellow yolk simply means that the hen has been fed a corn- rather than wheat-based diet, or has been fed a lot of yellow-orange plant pigments (xanthophylls). Because most consumers like their yolks nice and yellow, some poultry farmers add marigold petals to the diet of laying hens for this reason. Artificial color additives are not permitted. But be on a safety watch for albumen (white of the egg) that is pinkish or iridescent, since this could mean that it is contaminated with *Pseudomonas* bacteria. Even though this is not the worst bacteria to swallow, throw out the egg anyway. And what about that nasty green color that we sometimes see around the yolk of a boiled egg or as a tint to scrambled eggs? Eat away. It is not dangerous, though you may want to close your eyes so you don't see it. It is usually caused by overcooking, or cooking eggs at too high a temperature. If you are a frequent flier, you will have been served green scrambled eggs for an occasional in-flight breakfast. Unless you are starving, you may want to pass, but not because of health risks. They taste awful—even worse than most airline food.

Are fertile and double-yolk eggs safe?

It is rare to find a fertile egg in a carton these days, as roosters are usually not kept with laying hens. (I recall how that crowing rooster used to bother the neighbors, when we kept laying hens in our suburban backyard.) My mother used to believe that fertile eggs have special nutritional value, as many people do. There is no evidence for this. What you may get in fertilized eggs is a small amount of male hormone. But they are safe to eat. However, you need to remember that they do not keep as well as nonfertile eggs. As for double-yolk eggs, I was always told that if you found one, you would have good luck, although I offer no guarantees. And again, they are perfectly safe. A hen sometimes produces one near the beginning or end of its reproductive life. But if cooking with a double-yolk egg, you may want to adjust the number of eggs a bit to make extra allowances.

Are blood spots in eggs dangerous?

No, blood spots in eggs are not dangerous. They may look unappetizing, but you can eat them without any risk. Most people think that blood spots on egg yolk mean that the egg has been fertilized, but this is not true. Actually, they are caused by the rupture of a blood vessel or by a similar type of incident when the egg is being formed. Only about 1 percent of eggs have blood spots, and most of these eggs are eliminated before they reach the consumer. Blood spots are only found in fresh eggs, so in a way, you can look at it as a sign of freshness.

Can you ever get dangerous mold in eggs?

Molds such as *Penicillum, Rhizopus,* and *Alternaria* can indeed grow on the shell of eggs and even get inside if storage conditions are very moist. You may see them as powdery spots on the egg surface. Usually they are not dangerous. However, it *is* possible for the molds that produce the dangerous toxin aflatoxin (see page 54) to also contaminate eggs, although in the United States this occurs very rarely and is therefore not discussed in this chapter. However, in food safety, it is always better to assume that anything can happen.

How should eggs be stored at home?

How long eggs can be stored at home depends on what form the eggs are in and how they are being stored. The general rule is, "Keep eggs cold." Buy only refrigerated shell eggs, and at home, always keep in the main section of the refrigerator, not in the door. Do not wash USDA-graded eggs, as this will remove the protective mineral oil coating and allow bacteria to enter the egg more easily. If bought fresh and kept cool, eggs can be kept for three to five weeks after the date you purchase them. The sell-by date will probably expire during that time, but according to the FDA, CDC, and American Egg Board (which has a vested interest in making sure you don't get sick from your eggs), the eggs should still continue to be safe for a while afterward, depending on how this date relates to the pack-date. If the carton only has a date showing when the eggs were packed, you can keep them for four or five weeks after this date, as long as they are properly refrigerated. (See page 229 for more specific information.) Remember, too, that the faster you use those eggs, the less chance there will be for any bacteria in them to multiply.

How long do boiled eggs keep without spoiling?

Contrary to what most of us believe, hard-boiled eggs actually spoil faster than uncooked eggs, as the protective coating has been washed away and bacteria can enter the porous shell more easily. Cooked eggs should be refrigerated within two hours of cooking and eaten within one week. You may want to pass on that pile of boiled eggs sitting in a pretty bowl on top of the lunch counter or at the deli, unless you just saw someone take the bowl out of the refrigerator or the eggs out of the pot.

Which egg-containing foods are safest for pregnant women, young children, older adults or people with a compromised immune system?

When I was five years old, my most-hated food was raw eggs—which I was made to suck out of a shell with a hole at either end. I was told that this would help cure my anemia and asthma. I doubt many parents make their children do this nowadays, even in Europe. Amazingly, I survived—and the asthma did disappear, though I cannot claim that raw eggs were the cure. Actually, any food that is made with raw eggs or lightly cooked eggs falls into the "avoid" group of foods for those people at higher risk (see sidebar on page 6). If you are making these foods yourself, use pasteurized egg or pasteurized egg product or try heating the egg first (see next section). When eating any of these foods out, ask if raw shell egg is being used, and if the answer is yes, ask if the eggs are pasteurized. If not, order something else.

Smart Ways to Reduce Your Risks

ALTHOUGH SOME OF the material in this chapter may have destroyed your faith in the purity of the egg, it is really not that bad. Unlike several of the other foods discussed in this book, the consumer can do much to ensure that eggs are safe to eat. There is an easy solution for the main risks. It can be summed up as: "Keep cool and cook thoroughly."

Buy the freshest eggs possible. Buy eggs only from a refrigerated case (or, in a farmers' market, those kept in a cooler). Always purchase eggs or egg products before the sell-by or expiration date on the carton, if there is such a date (you may have trouble finding it, especially if you live in a state that forbids such dates). If not, look at the packing date and make sure it was no more than a couple of weeks ago. When choosing a container of liquid egg product, also check the date, and make sure the carton is tightly sealed and not swollen.

Buy the safest eggs possible. The USDA grade mark on egg cartons has safety value, as it tells you that the plant that processed the eggs is following the good manufacturing and sanitation practices advised by the USDA. If you buy your eggs at a farmers' market or a small store, remember that current (as of 2010) government safety regulations do not apply to producers with fewer than three thousand laying hens or to producers who sell all of their eggs directly to consumers. This does not mean that such eggs are unsafe. But it puts more responsibility on you—the buyer—to make sure they are. Talk to the vendor.

Wherever you are buying, open the carton to make sure the eggs inside are uncracked (gently spin each in its compartment; a badly cracked egg will stick). If you are particularly anxious to avoid eggs produced by hens that have received antibiotics, buy organic or labeled "antibiotic free." Some studies have found that chickens that have recently been given antibiotics produce eggs with thinner shells, but dietary factors can produce the same results. If you want extra safety, or plan to make eggs or dishes in which eggs will remain undercooked, then buy pasteurized shell eggs or pasteurized egg product. Hen welfare issues have not been proven to have safety benefits.

Use eggs carefully. It is smart to simply assume that the egg inside the shell could be contaminated with bacteria (even though this is not very likely if you have followed the above purchasing advice). Therefore, avoid cross-contamination of raw eggs with other foods, and wash your hands after touching raw egg. Don't take eggs out of the refrigerator more than two hours before you are ready to use them. If you accidentally crack a raw egg, use it immediately or (if you only notice it later) discard it.

Cook eggs thoroughly. Both the whites and the yolk should be firm (not soft). If you like your omelets soft, use pasteurized eggs or egg product. If you use a food thermometer, you can assume that egg whites will coagulate at 144°–149°F, egg yolks at 149°–158°F, and whole eggs at 144°–158°F. Let's say that 160°F is a safe internal temperature to aim for. If a hard-boiled egg cracks during cooking, it should be safe to eat. Dry meringue is safe, as are meringue-topped pies if they are cooked to 350°F for about 15 minutes. However, desserts such as chiffon pies could be unsafe. Serve dishes that contain eggs as soon as they are ready, or refrigerate, to avoid their picking up contaminants.

Take special measures when making dishes that contain raw or undercooked eggs. If you are making foods such as mayonnaise or ice cream at home from scratch, use pasteurized eggs or pasteurized egg product. The USDA suggests a way to make such recipes safe with regular shell eggs, but it is a bit tricky: Try heating the eggs in a liquid from the recipe over low heat, stirring constantly, until the mixture reaches 160°F, and keep at that temperature for a few seconds. Then combine it with the other ingredients and complete the recipe. If you want to prepare an egg-containing dish ahead of time (I have several great ones that I like to whip out for company), cook it within 24 hours of serving and keep it refrigerated.

Keep eggs, egg products, and egg dishes cold and don't store too long. Keep eggs in the main section of the refrigerator (not the door) at no higher a temperature than 45°F. Pasteurized eggs have to be stored the same way as unpasteurized raw eggs. Keep whole eggs in their carton, or place them in another closed container and tear off and keep their expiry date with the eggs. (Before I started doing this, I used to often come home from a trip, unable to remember when I bought the eggs that I found sitting there.) Keeping eggs in their carton or other container may also prevent them from absorbing any strong odors from foods. See the chart for specific guidance about egg storage, based on USDA data.

. . .

EGG STORAGE RECOMMENDATIONS

Egg Product	Stored in Refrigerator (on shelves)	Stored in Freezer
Raw eggs	In shell, 3–5 weeks	Do not freeze.
	Egg yolks only, 2–4 days	12 months
	Whites only, 2–4 days	Do not freeze well
Hard-cooked eggs	1 week	Do not freeze.
Egg substitutes, liquid	Unopened, 10 days Opened, 3 days	Do not freeze.
Egg substitutes, frozen	Unopened, after thawing, 7 days, or refer to use-by date on carton Opened, 3 days, or refer to use-by date on the carton	12 months
Casseroles made with eggs	3–4 days	After baking, 2–3 months
Eggnog	Commercial, 3–5 days	6 months
	Homemade, 2-4 days	Do not freeze
Pies	Pumpkin or pecan, 3–4 days	After baking, 1 –2 months
	Custard or chiffon, 3-4 days	Do not freeze.
Quiche with any kind of filling	3–4 days	After baking, 1–2 months

Don't taste foods containing raw egg. As mentioned earlier (and see also sidebar, page 246), this is something to watch when preparing cookie dough, cake batter, or puddings (even as I write this, I am embarrassed to say that I wasn't very good at stopping my own son from licking the spoon). Ignore recipe instructions to add seasonings "to taste" if a mixture (such as a pasta filling) contains raw egg.

Be even more careful when eating eggs at restaurants or overseas. Be extra careful to avoid undercooked egg dishes when eating outside your home. Simply don't order sunny-side up or soft-boiled eggs, soft omelets, or even eggs Benedict, and pass up egg-based dressings, unless you are told that pasteurized eggs or egg product is being used. As for some of those wonderful desserts that may contain raw egg—make sure that pasteurized or processed eggs have been used. When eating in-flight breakfasts, don't eat the egg if it smells odd (you would be surprised at how many people have contracted food poisoning on a plane).

9

Grains, Legumes, and Nuts

ARSENIC TURNING UP in rice? The government telling Americans that alfalfa is too dangerous to eat? Huge outbreaks involving peanuts? Microbes getting right inside nut shells? Toxic mold risks everywhere? We don't think of grains, legumes, or nuts as particularly risky foods. But at times they can be. Even in North America. The smart thing to do—as usual—is to know when they're unsafe for us, and either avoid eating them, or know how to reduce the risks.

The following pages will again bring out some of the main themes of this book: A food that is healthy from a nutritional point of view is not always healthy from a safety one. (Rice bran could prove to be one of those that aren't.) Our industrialized food supply is spreading risks, including when grains, legumes, and nuts are comingled in huge storage facilities. Raw is riskier—as with raw sprouted seeds and raw nuts. There can also be trade-offs in avoiding one type of safety risk and avoiding another, as when we have to choose between the possible risk of bacteria or pesticide residue in your raw nuts. Similarly to the other foods we have looked at in earlier chapters, we often can't tell by appearance if a grain, nut, or legume is contaminated. And, as usual, there are also so many contradictory research findings and views, so much we still don't know. There is always that long-term study gap. Which—again, as always—leaves us having to rely on the information we do have and our own judgment, until we know more.

What We Eat

ALMOST EVERYONE IN North America eats at least some grains and legumes, although perhaps not tree nuts. But again, as we saw in discussions of produce, meat, dairy, and eggs, our preferences are shifting.

Grains

Foods made from grains are an important part of our diet—perhaps too important in the United States and Canada. But we may not be eating the same grains our parents or grandparents did. For one thing, North Americans are eating less wheat and more rice—about twice as much rice as we ate ten years ago. We eat the wheat mainly in the form of yeast breads and rolls, quick breads, and other baked goods made from flour. Corn remains popular in our breakfast cereals and in many popular snacks, such as popcorn and corn chips. Oats are also still a favorite breakfast food for us (as well as for our horses, cattle, chickens, and dogs). The most rapid growth in breakfast cereals, by the way, has been in RTE cereals. As always, we are willing to pay a premium for any ready-to-eat food that saves us a few minutes of time.

Usually we eat wheat flour, rice, and rice products as highly processed grains, with most of the nutrients removed. But since the 1970s, other more exotic grains, including many whole grains, are increasingly catching on. Who doesn't want to eat something that might just help reduce their risk of type 2 diabetes, cardiovascular disease, cancer—and, perhaps just as important—the risk of getting fat! The government has advised us to eat at least three servings of whole grains a day. The food industry has happily gone along.

Legumes

Legumes have a superhealthy image. We have hundreds of varieties of legumes to choose from, including beans, lentils, peas, soy, peanuts, alfalfa, and clover. And we can feel righteous eating them because they are such a high source of protein. One cup of black beans is claimed to provide about as much protein as three ounces of broiled steak. But most Americans would rather choose the steak than the beans, wrongly believing that proteins should come from meat, fish, and dairy. USDA Dietary Guidelines recommend that we eat six servings (three cups) of legumes a week if our overall calorie intake is around 2,000 kcal/day. But most of us don't eat enough of them. Peanuts—which we wrongly tend to think of as a "nut"—are America's favorite legume, and peanut butter is our favorite peanut food.

Tree Nuts

Tree nuts include almonds, cashews, coconut, macadamia nuts, pecans, pine nuts, pistachios, walnuts, and more unusual ones such as acorns, beech nuts, and tiger nuts. In North America, you are either a tree nut eater or you are not. Some reports say that only one in ten Americans eats them, averaging out to about 3.4 pounds of tree nuts per person per year. (As someone who eats a handful of walnuts or pecans on top of fruit every morning, I am certainly warping those statistics.) Tree nuts are not nearly as popular as peanuts. But in spite of this, in the United States, people are eating more tree nuts today than in the 1990s. Canadians, too, are apparently increasing their nut consumption, particularly in the form of trail mix. Almonds are our most popular tree nut, accounting for about a third of the tree nuts we eat. Next in line are those other nuts, such as cashews, walnuts, and pecans, followed by hazelnuts and pistachios.

Who Keeps It Safe?

IN THE UNITED States, the FDA is in charge of making sure that legumes, grains, and nuts and products derived from them, are safe, wholesome, and properly labeled. Other federal agencies, state agencies, and industry organizations are also involved. The FDA's responsibilities include the usual things, such as issuing safety guidance to the industry, inspecting plant facilities, labeling, and maintaining oversight of any recalls. In Canada, the responsible agencies are again the HC and CFIA. The industries are active through their respective organizations.

Government is progressively trying to improve safety of these foods, although they may not have as high priority as some others. Often a new push for new safety measures or higher standards has followed a public outcry that has followed an outbreak. For instance, when several outbreaks of bacteria in raw sprouts underlined safety risks, the FDA issued safety guidance to the American sprout producers and distributors. After the 2009 large peanut, and later, pistachio product–associated outbreaks, the FDA provided the peanut industry, and then the nut industry, with special guidance on how to avoid *Salmonella* bacteria.

The problem, of course, is that the guidance is not binding. Basically, it is up to the grower or plant operator to apply best practices—and to government inspections to catch them if they don't. As always, there are too few inspectors, too little money for thorough inspections, and companies that put profits far above public safety. Some processing plants may only be inspected once every four years—and even then, just given a quick look-see. No inspector wanted to find problems, which usually means they have to take test samples and then follow up. The easiest solution, and the one that pleases everyone, is just to give a nice positive report—while the contaminated grain, legume, or nut and its products continue to be released into the marketplace.

Nor is it easy for the government to take tough action against the industry, even if warranted. In one recently reported case of a thirty-year-old company that distributed tainted alfalfa to multiple states, the FDA issued repeated warnings about poor sanitary conditions. After about nine years of these, during which the company reportedly did not comply and kept on putting out some five hundred pounds of product a day, the FDA finally issued a permanent injunction. In the meantime, we kept eating the alfalfa.

Industry associations wield considerable political power. This can operate for, or against, greater safety. The National Grain and Feed Association (NFGA), which handles over two thirds of all U.S. grains and oilseeds, and the Almond Board of California (ABC) are two such industry bodies. Although we consumers tend to think of the industry as fighting stricter safety measures, it can be the reverse. ABC's role in promoting the sterilization of raw nuts (after costly outbreaks associated with almonds in 2004) is an example. ABC also worked with nut growers and processors to encourage them to use safer practices. But the bottom line is that it is all about the "bottom line"—profits.

Again, our industrialized food supply complicates safety oversight. In the case of grains, nuts, and some legumes—as with fruits and vegetables, eggs, dairy, and other foods—commingling of product from several farms can spread contaminants from one to the other. Cereal crops from different sources are mixed together upon receipt by the grain elevator, and sometimes even earlier, when one farm does the milling for neighboring farms. Or they are mixed during trucking to the elevator. The U.S. Bioterrorism Act of 2002 partly addressed this issue, requiring facilities to register with the FDA. New legislation under the Food Safety Modernization Act (pending at the time of publication) would increase preventive controls to address some of the risks created by the comingling of these foods. This is not being welcomed by many in the industry because it adds to paperwork and operating costs. Unfortunately, as often happens, the smaller producers are likely to find such measures most difficult.

Battling Microbes in Legumes and Tree Nuts

WE DON'T NORMALLY think of bacteria or viruses in connection with grains, legumes, or nuts. But don't dismiss the idea yet. These days, that hardy *Salmonella* family of bugs is everywhere. Remember the widespread outbreaks of *Salmonella* bacteria associated with peanuts (a legume) in 2008 and pistachios (a tree nut) in 2009? And did you know that the frequency of bacterial contamination of alfalfa (which is actually a legume) makes it one of the most dangerous raw foods you can eat?

In the 1960s and '70s, the free-spirited hippie generation popularized sprouting legume seeds, such as mung bean, cress, clover, and alfalfa. Even a few decades ago, I—and almost everyone I knew in Washington, D.C.—grew sprouts at home. We ate them on our sandwiches, salads, and soups because we thought they were superhealthy. Now the FDA is warning us to avoid them—even the home-grown ones (see sidebar).

FDA ADVICE TO CONSUMERS ON THE HEALTH RISKS OF RAW SPROUTS

Raw sprouts that are served on salads, wraps, and sandwiches may contain bacteria that can cause food-borne illness. Rinsing sprouts first will not remove bacteria. Home-grown sprouts also present a health risk if they are eaten raw or lightly cooked.

◇ To reduce the risk of illness, do not eat raw sprouts such as bean, alfalfa, clover, or radish sprouts. All sprouts should be cooked thoroughly before eating to reduce the risk of illness.

◇ This advice is particularly important for children, the
   elderly, and persons with weakened immune systems,
   all of whom are at risk of developing serious illness due
   to food-borne disease.

SOURCE: http://www.fda.gov/downloads/Food/ResourcesForYou/
Consumers/UCM174142.pdf

Health Canada as well as the FDA have warned consumers not to
eat raw sprouted seeds. In fact, Health Canada suggests that you
don't even *touch* raw sprouts. Sprouted seeds have been contaminated
just too many times with dangerous bacteria such as various *Salmonella* spp., *E. coli* O157:H7, and even *Listeria monocytogenes*. Over a
period of ten years, I found an average of about three recorded outbreaks a year in America, and outbreaks are still occurring as I write.
In one case there were *four* kinds of *Salmonella* bacteria involved in
just one contaminated seed lot. During just the first five months of
2009, there was an outbreak of *Salmonella saintpaul* in alfalfa and of
Listeria monocytogenes in bean and soy sprouts, which is more unusual.
The alfalfa one was relatively large by sprout standards, causing over
230 illnesses in fourteen states; the *Salmonella*-contaminated seeds
had been distributed to U.S. growers nationwide. It was virtually
impossible to find sprouts that *weren't* likely to be contaminated. In
fact, in April 2009, the FDA and CDC suggested that *no one* in the
United States—even healthy adults—eat raw alfalfa sprouts, or eat
any blends containing alfalfa, until further notice. But well into the
recall, I found several of my neighborhood stores were still selling
alfalfa without posting any warning notice. Consumer beware!

Once sprouts have become infected, there is really no solution
apart from cooking them—as advised by the FDA. Washing
doesn't help because, usually, the bacteria are right inside the seed.

Seed distributors believe that the bacteria enter in the field, as a
result of improperly composted manure used as fertilizer, from
grazing animals, or from contaminated irrigation water. Or they
enter in seed silos from bird or mouse droppings or urine. Mice

and cockroaches running around the alfalfa plant can be a hazard, too (That was one of the problems at the alfalfa plant mentioned earlier). Is this enough to make you stop eating raw sprouts?

Although there may be very few bacteria present initially in a sprout seed, they multiply rapidly under those nice warm and moist sprouting conditions. In a few days they can increase to millions of bacteria per serving. It could well be that the chances of getting ill from that tiny mound of sprouts on top of your salad are greater than from the plate of lettuce underneath. In fact, more outbreaks have been associated with sprouts than with juice, berries, tomatoes, or melons. The number of people affected is relatively small because most North Americans don't eat sprouts. Usually the culprit sprout has been alfalfa, as it is the most popular one we eat.

Government and industry *have* been working on ways to make sprouts less risky. But either some growers are not following the FDA guidance (such as seed disinfection prior to growing), or the procedures are not working as they should. Nor are we consumers always following warnings. Those who became ill during the 2009 outbreak in alfalfa ranged from less than twelve months to eighty-five years old. Both ends of this age spectrum fall into high-risk groups that the FDA advises *never* to eat raw sprouts—even when there is no known outbreak ongoing.

Let's take a look at microbes in another, much more popular legume—peanuts. Whereas only about 8 percent of the U.S. population eats alfalfa, almost every American household buys peanuts or peanut products or both. Along with beans and lentils, peanuts, too, are claimed to be very good for us. Various studies tout various health benefits of peanuts, ranging from improved circulation and brain health to reduction of cancer risks and cardiovascular disease. It has even been claimed—but not yet proven for humans—that peanuts slow aging (they supposedly contain more resveratrol than do grapes) and reduce impotence. Not bad.

According the National Peanut Board, we consume an average six pounds of peanuts and three and a half pounds of peanut butter per year. The average American child will eat more than fifteen hundred peanut butter and jelly sandwiches before he or she graduates from high school. We also use peanut ingredients in a myriad of other processed foods. That is part of the problem. If a microbe contaminates an ingredient that is used by hundreds of food manufacturers, illnesses can spread far and wide and be very difficult to trace (as we also saw in the case of milk ingredients). Companies that use peanuts or peanut ingredients can become innocent victims of an unethical—or sometimes, just plain careless—peanut product supplier. This is what happened in the two large peanut-associated outbreaks of 2007 and 2009 (see sidebar).

TWO MAJOR SCANDALS STARTED BY A SMALL "NUT"

In 2007 *Salmonella tennessee* bacteria contaminated Peter Pan and Super Value peanut butter. Over 600 people from forty-seven states were sickened, with four unconfirmed deaths. The bacteria were traced to a ConAgra plant in Sylvester, Georgia. In 2008–2009, there was another and even larger peanut-related outbreak, caused by another Salmonella bacteria (*S. Typhimurium*). It originated in a Blakely, Georgia, processing plant, operated by the Peanut Corporation of America (PCA), located only seventy-five miles from where the 2007 outbreak started.

PCA was an unethical company, running a cut-rate operation to maximize profits, with little importance given to its clients' interests or to consumer safety. This company distributed its products to at least one thousand other large and small companies, which used the peanuts as an ingredient in twenty-one hundred other foods, such as cereals, snack bars, candy, chocolates, cookies, ice cream, pies, cakes, frozen dinners, and even pet food. At least 714 people (and many dogs) became ill in forty-six states, with nine suspected deaths. The real numbers of victims are always many times higher than those reported. In the 2008–2009 case, which I followed closely, the illnesses continued for almost a year afterward. Many of the contaminated products—such as peanut butter crackers—have a long shelf life, and people did not pay attention to the recall.

In both these peanut-related cases, the peanut-supplier companies involved had found *Salmonella* to be present in their products many times during their own testing (twelve times in the later outbreak). In spite of this, they released products into the marketplace. In both instances, overloaded inspectors had given the plants high marks for safety. (The reports are an amazing read.) After the outbreaks, federal inspectors took a more careful look. They found dangerous processing and storage conditions behind both outbreaks—problems such as a leaky roof and faulty sprinkler head that caused heavy moisture, poor in-plant sanitation, risky storage of raw peanuts and peanut product next to each other, poor equipment maintenance and quality control, and insects flying or running around all over the place—in other words, just about everything we would hope to never find in a place where food is made.

Such outbreaks are a nightmare for everyone. After the truth came out, PCA closed down its plants and filed for bankruptcy, leaving the poor underfunded and overworked FDA and state agencies to deal with the mess. Several "downstream" companies were forced to file for Chapter 11 bankruptcy. Food banks had to throw out masses of food, at a time when they were struggling to meet the increasing demand created by the recession.

But in all this, it was the children who suffered most. In the case of both peanut-related outbreaks, they were more than half the victims.

Can *roasted* peanuts also be contaminated? Unfortunately, yes, although less frequently. Peanuts come out of the ground covered in dirt, and let's face it, we all know that dirt is "dirty." In fact, soil is loaded with different kinds of bacteria, some harmless to humans, some dangerous. The worst ones, like the more toxic *E. coli* and some in the *Salmonella* family, usually get into the soil from animal or human feces. Peanuts can pick up these bacteria, which can even get under the shells. They can stay there, while the peanut plants are mechanically harvested, dried in the sun for a few days, and the peanuts are separated from their vines and then air-dried. Even if roasting does kill most of these bacteria, the few tougher ones left will multiply. New ones can also enter at later points, as we also saw with other foods. Also, as mentioned earlier, recent studies are showing that *Salmonella* bacteria can be quite heat resistant, and even thrive under dry conditions (see also the following chapter).

And what about tree nuts such as almonds, walnuts, pecans, pistachios, and others? Yes, these nuts grow up high on trees—not in the soil. But they can also be contaminated with bacteria, although outbreaks linked to such nuts are relatively infrequent. However, a large recall of pistachios and pistachio products did occur in 2009. Some tests found *Salmonella* bacteria. Others did not. But ultimately 664 pistachio, as well as pistachio-containing products, were recalled—snack bars, cakes, candies, snack foods, and ice creams. And wouldn't you know it—it was discovered that one of the client companies, which had been forced to recall its packaged pistachios, sent them right back into the food supply with a new healthy-sounding label and new packaging.

A few outbreaks have also been associated with almonds, which are a more popular nut in North America than pistachios. In 2004, an outbreak of *Salmonella* bacteria in California-grown raw almonds caused dozens of illnesses in several countries. In the United States, the almonds had been packaged and sold under several well-known brands and in such large retail outlets as Costco and Trader Joe's. Some eighteen million pounds of almonds had to be recalled.

Some of the outbreaks of bacteria in tree nuts originate at the grower level (such as when fallen nuts are mixed into the supply), some during storage, transport, or processing. As with peanuts, there are a number of windows of opportunity for bacteria to get in. That 2004 contamination of almonds by *Salmonella* was traced back to two contaminated huller-shellers used by one of California's largest almond producers. Also, bacteria may even survive peanut and nut treatment with chlorine solution, drying, and roasting at high temperatures. Because of the industrialized nature of our food supply, a few bad nuts can contaminate many, many more—here, too, mixing increases risks. And because nuts are such a common ingredient in so many manufactured foods, problems spread.

Battling Microbes in Grain-Based Foods

LET'S TURN BRIEFLY to microbes in foods based on grains such as wheat, rice, oats, barley, quinoa, and so on. There have been several significant cases of microbe contamination of grain-based processed foods over the years—breads and bakery goods and even cereals. Often some other ingredient is to blame, or some other factor, rather than the grain itself. The Center for Science in the Public Interest (CSPI) lists 179 small and larger outbreaks in these foods between 1997 and 2006, most of which were caused by viruses, not bacteria—especially the very contagious norovirus. But *Salmonella* spp. bacteria have a strong lead over others for second place. Bacteria such as *Staphylococcus aureus, Clostridium perfringens, Listeria monocytogenes,* and *Bacillus cereus* have also cropped up from time to time.

The greater majority of safety problems that have occurred with baked goods happened in institutional settings (such as schools, nursing homes, jails, and country clubs), at receptions and other large social gatherings (weddings, church socials, and so on), and in delis or restaurants. Let me tell you about a personal experience that happened just a few days ago. It occurred in a charming Italian restaurant in Berkeley, California. From where we sat, we could see the maître d' showing a waitress how to turn two precut slices of chocolate cake into a birthday cake for a customer. First, he used his bare (unwashed) hands to lift the cake slices onto a plate (just before that, we had seen him handle cash and other objects, and he had also shaken hands with a customer). Then he joined them together by wetting his index finger (no, no glove) and using it to smear the icing across, so that the join was invisible. Then the waitress, who had just a moment ago sneezed and correctly covered her mouth, got into the act, using her bare hands to improve the join around the edges. Finally, the candle that had been sitting on the counter was placed in the middle of the cake. In just a couple of minutes they had broken a number of basic restaurant hygiene rules—and put the diner at risk.

As it happens, chocolate cake is one of the most common causes of bakery-related illnesses, along with coconut cream and other cream pies. They are popular with microbes as well as us. Poor hygiene among food-service workers is a common cause. My experience was not that unusual.

But occasionally cereals can also become contaminated by bacteria during processing, resulting in much larger outbreaks. Often it is *Salmonella* bacteria again. Contaminated processing equipment was found to be a culprit in a thirty-state outbreak of *Salmonella agona* in toasted oat cereal several years ago, with at least 215 confirmed illnesses. An investigation into an outbreak of another *Salmonella* in infant cereal found that it had been adulterated with "cleaning remains" from milling machinery. When infant foods are contaminated, things really become frightening.

We consumers can also be responsible for problems. When microwaving baked goods such as meat pies, we don't always take uneven microwave heating into account, resulting in inadequate cooking. That is apparently what happened in a 2007 incident involving *Salmonella* in chicken pot pies, which made at least 139 Americans ill in thirty states. And then there is cookie dough. The media and politicians were up in arms when *E. coli* O157:H7 was discovered in packaged raw dough in 2009 (see sidebar).

RAW AND RISKY COOKIE DOUGH

You don't need to be a child to love raw cookie dough. These days, with Americans everywhere looking for time- and mess-saving shortcuts, ready-to-bake cookie dough is a welcome solution. Open the refrigerated package and pop the dough into the oven—that's all it takes. This is even faster than my three-minute homemade peanut-butter cookie recipe. That is, if the dough is not eaten before it ever reaches that cookie sheet.

In mid-2009 we learned to our horror that Nestlé's packaged Toll House Cookie Dough—one of the most popular brands—was accused by the FDA of being contaminated with *E. coli* O157:H7 bacteria. At least eighty related illnesses were reported in thirty-one states. Symptoms (diarrhea, abdominal pain, vomiting) started from one to eight days after the tainted dough was eaten raw. Most healthy adults recovered within a week.

No surprise, about 65 percent of those who became ill were two to nineteen years old—at the age when raw cookie dough is the most tempting. Young children and the elderly were at highest risk of ending up in hospital. Almost thirty did, several with a type of kidney failure called hemolytic uremic syndrome (HUS). But healthy adults can also become seriously ill, as in the case of one woman who had to have her gall bladder and part of her colon removed, lost her speech, and spent at least 120 days in the hospital. One four-year-old girl suffered a stroke and remains partially paralyzed. These are just two of the tragic stories.

The FDA and CDC warned consumers to throw out the dough, and not even to bake it, because even handling it could prove dangerous. Nestlé recalled some three hundred thousand cases of the product although the company did not fully accept that their dough was to blame, and its own routine testing for bacteria had turned up nothing. Nestlé nevertheless did a thorough testing of its facility, production equipment, processes, ingredients, and finished product to try to locate the cause. It bought new eggs, flour, and margarine before restarting production several months later. The product now carries a large label warning against eating raw dough. There goes another of life's pleasures. But I have noticed that although Nestlé dough now carries such clear warnings, other brands of similar cookie dough product sitting right next to them in our supermarket aisle do not. The risk in eating those is just as great.

Getting Serious About Mold Toxins

You MAY RECALL aflatoxin from discussions of mold in previous chapters. Currently, researchers concur that aflatoxin B1 (AFB1) is the worst mycotoxin that molds can produce in our food. It is the most potent natural carcinogen known. This, and other aflatoxins, are frequently present in grains, peanuts, nuts, and other foods. But they are not the only ones. Other mold toxins—such as vomitoxins and fumonisins—are also common in grains, peanuts, and tree nuts.

Let's get down to the specifics. Among the most hazardous foods for such mold toxins are:

- **Grains**—especially corn, wheat, pearl millet, rice, and sorghum
- **Legumes**—such as peanuts, peanut products, and soybeans
- **Tree nuts**—such as almonds, pistachios, walnuts, and coconuts

The industry does try to keep levels of these mycotoxins low, for purely economic reasons if nothing else. It has been estimated that the presence of such toxins can cause losses as great as two billion dollars per year in U.S. grain commodities. The government also tries to keep levels low in our nuts, at least taking action if the aflatoxin levels in pistachio and Brazil nuts, and in peanuts and peanut products, go above 20 ppb. But keeping mold toxins out is far from easy.

Studies have shown that, while growing, such foods tend to become contaminated with toxin-producing molds when climatic and soil conditions are favorable (and who can control the weather?). Molds can also be encouraged by poor harvesting practices and storage under hot and moist conditions. Insects help. In the case of peanuts or tree nuts, toxin-producing fungi get right inside if there are breaks in the protective layer of the nut through which the burrowing insects, carrying fungal spores, can enter. Over the years, insects have been developing greater resistance to approved pesticides. And a contaminated peanut or tree nut cannot always be eliminated from the load of nuts sent to market, because growers often cannot tell by looking at a nut that fungi are in it. Testing does not catch every contaminated grain or nut, either.

There are two basic ways that the more dangerous aflatoxins (and other mycotoxins) in nuts, legumes, or grains could affect us. We could get a case of acute aflatoxosis (with symptoms such as liver damage, hemorrhage, and various digestive problems, which can be fatal). Or, over a period of years, small but regular amounts of mold toxins can leave us with certain vague digestive and other health issues. These latter symptoms are very difficult to identify, and are often wrongly diagnosed.

Before you get too worried—acute cases of aflatoxosis are very rare in North America. The only relatively large outbreak I came across—more correctly, a series of outbreaks—with a *possible* (note the qualification) mycotoxin cause, were certainly both puzzling and frightening. These incidents were linked to wheat burritos in the school lunch program. During twelve months in 1997–1998, there were sixteen separate incidents in Pennsylvania, Kansas, Florida, Georgia, Illinois, Indiana, and North Dakota. An estimated nineteen hundred people (mostly children, of course) became ill. Often as quickly as only thirty minutes after eating the school lunch, they came down with gastrointestinal problems and neurological symptoms such as headache, dizziness, and tingling or burning of the mouth. (Imagine the scene in the schools). Oddly enough, ten very similar outbreaks occurred in 2003–2004 in nine different Massachusetts schools. So much for that nice, "healthy" school lunch.

Although we don't need to be greatly concerned about sudden mycotoxin-caused illnesses in North America, chronic exposure could be a different matter. The FDA considers aflatoxins to be "unavoidable food contaminants." The agency does try to control the amounts that are present and hope that not too many of us build up sufficient quantities to notice. We can assume that we are getting small amounts of aflatoxins, and other mold toxins, from several of our food items every day. For that reason, the United States and Canada—along with hundreds of other countries—have established "maximum acceptable levels" in our foods. Anything at this level or below can enter the marketplace. If it is above it, the government will take action. Up to a point, this is fine. But there are three issues that worry me.

One is that we are allowing much higher levels of such toxins in our food than do most other countries. The levels of aflatoxins considered safe in North America are 20 ppb (except for milk, which is lower), whereas in Europe and some most other countries the ceiling is 4 ppb. Are we really tougher than the French, Swedes, or Germans?

Another troubling issue is the practical difficulty of actually keeping higher-than-permitted levels of such mycotoxins out of our food supply. This is very dependent on getting a good sample for testing. But the levels of toxin in a truckload of, say, raw peanuts, or grains stored in an elevator, will vary from one part of the contents to another (probably more so, because of commingling). Tests do not always take a composite sample or sample periodically from a moving stream of grains or nuts. I have found reports on testing of U.S.-grown peanuts in warehouses where over 50 percent turned up levels that were almost *twice* as high as allowed. That doesn't mean it happens all the time, but it *can* happen. Some food safety experts have also pointed out that there is no measurement of aflatoxin levels *after* products such as peanut butter reach the stores. It is possible that the levels may have increased. Molds can be right there in the jar, happily spitting out toxins, and the purchaser may not even see or taste them.

My third concern: These levels are set according to how much the government estimates the riskiest foods might turn up in an *average* diet. What if your child or mine regularly eats more than that base number of peanut butter and jelly sandwiches, and does it over a period of years? What if you follow a vegetarian or vegan diet that relies more heavily on grains, nuts, and legumes for protein? Or what if you eat a high-corn diet, as many Mexican Americans do? And what if you are getting regular doses of these foods from several sources at once, as in the case of someone who eats a lot of corn-based foods *and* peanuts and peanut-butter?

As usual, vulnerability has a lot to do with our risk, and here again those in high-risk groups, such as children or people with other health conditions, are among the most vulnerable. An illustration: Several studies have even found that aflatoxins and the hepatitis B virus act as "cocarcinogens." This means that if you are one of the millions of people in North America who are living with chronic hepatitis B (an estimated forty-three hundred new cases of it are diagnosed every year in the United States, with a very high incidence in some cities, such as San Francisco)—you are something like twelve times more likely to develop liver cancer if you are *also* exposed to certain aflatoxins. How this happens is too complex to get into here . . . but has your doctor even warned you about the mold connection?

There may also be synergy between aflatoxins and other myco-toxins, such as the aforementioned and aptly named vomitoxins and fumonisins. In some years, as much as half of the red winter wheat in certain parts of the United States has been badly contaminated with vomitoxin. Fumonisins are most likely to be present in corn and processed corn products; high levels have been found in some of the corn grown in Texas and Kentucky. At present, we know far less about fumonisins than we do about aflatoxins—but the news so far is *not* good. The IARC has classified some fumonisins as possibly human carcinogens (particularly as regards esophageal and liver cancer). The FDA is still trying to decide. If you are getting doses of these other mycotoxins as well as of aflatoxins—as can happen—conceivably the combined effect could be worse than any single one alone. This could put at risk people who eat large quantities of food such as corn tortillas—as some do—through regular exposure to aflatoxins as well as fumonisins. Research needs to study such issues more.

Now you see why, earlier, I said that I was more worried about mold in my food than in my house. What we do know about these fungi is largely negative—and there is so much more about these toxins that we still don't know.

The Pesticide Dilemma

PESTICIDES ARE COMMONLY used in production of grains, legumes, and tree nuts, both while growing in the field and during storage. Yes, such pesticides are used for good reason. Often that reason is insect control—including of those same insects that carry spores of the molds that produce the dangerous toxins we just looked at. Stored grains and nuts in bins and elevators, or even in the shop, can easily attract pests, particularly if they are kept for a long period of time in damp conditions. Wheat, corn, oats, barley, sorghum, kaffir seed, buckwheat, and other grains are all susceptible to insects such as weevils. Nuts can also attract a variety of insects, including maggots, weevils, caterpillars, webworms, stinkbugs, shuckworms, and spittlebugs (I love these names).

For the farmer or distributor, such freeloaders are bad news. To prevent these pests destroying their product and their profits, producers may apply a protective layer of an insecticide. If the pests are already there, fumigation (the exposure to toxic fumes) may be employed. The good news is that here in North America, such dangerous agricultural chemicals are strictly regulated. Only a few fumigants are approved for use where grain or nuts are stored. A skull-and-crossbones on the label reminds users of their dangers, and specific instructions are spelled out. But that does not mean that every farm or warehouse worker can follow (or even, read) those instructions. Nor does it mean that those approved pesticides are safe. The use of propylene oxide (PPO) to fumigate raw nuts is a case in point (see sidebar).

SAFETY TRADE-OFFS

The two relatively small but costly outbreaks of *Salmonella* bacteria in almonds in 2001 and 2004 were viewed as a major crisis by the California almond industry. Not wanting repeat performances, which could undermine almond producers' profits, the Almond Board of California (ABC) took action. It persuaded the USDA to legislate that all raw almonds sold in North America had to be either pasteurized by quick steaming of the nuts, or sprayed with the insecticide propylene oxide to kill any bacteria.

In theory, this sounds like a good idea. We are now less likely to get a case of *Salmonella* from our almonds. But of course, now we are likely to get PPO residues in their place. The IARC considers PPO to be a "possible" human carcinogen. EPA has classified it as a "Group B2, *probable* human carcinogen." Experiments with feeding it to mice and rats have found it to be "moderately toxic." Long-term exposure to small quantities of PPO may not have the drastic effects that massive exposure has. However, there is a possibility that it might gradually result in some neurological damage.

True, PPO may not be as toxic as some other pesticides that it has replaced, and it has been in use for years for spraying nuts in California. But PPO treatment of food is banned by the EU and several other countries, including Mexico and Canada, on grounds that it may harm human health. The ABC naturally argues that it is good because it helps to not only reduce bacteria, yeasts, and mold on nuts, but also control insects—all in one quick zap. And, it does not ruin the taste or texture of nuts, so consumers won't notice. Both the ABC and the FDA argue that PPO is perfectly safe for nuts that are consumed raw.

What about the alternative steam treatment? Yes, that avoids the risk of your raw almonds' giving you a dose of PPO. But the problem is that this treatment leaves "raw" almonds not really "raw" anymore, because they have been exposed to high heat. This bothers people on a raw diet. Some also say they don't taste as good. I have been looking for labels on raw nut bags to tell me which treatment has

> been used, but haven't found any. Store management hasn't been able to tell me, either. So what can we do if we don't want PPO, *and* don't want our "raw" almonds to really be cooked almonds? Well, we could always buy organic ones. But they will cost us more.

Let's turn to imports. Toxic pesticides, such as Aldrin and dieldrin, are reported to still be in use for killing insects around stored grains in some of the countries from which we import some nuts and grains. Dieldrin is considered a probable human carcinogen by the EPA and believed also to affect the immune system, and in high levels, the central nervous system. Some of the research I reviewed found that when pesticides containing dieldrin are sprayed on flour, corn, or other grain sacks, the pesticides give off a toxic vapor that can pass through jute materials of sacks, right into the contents. This can result in high toxin levels in the product inside.

Keeping Light on Heavy Metals

IN INDUSTRIAL SOCIETIES, heavy metals are everywhere. We pick them up from our water, air, soil—and our food. How well our body can deal with excess toxic metals seems to depend on a combination of factors that we can do nothing about—such as genetics, race, and how well our kidneys and digestive system are functioning. As usual, some of us are more at risk than others.

Grains can be a source of heavy metals. That is why the FDA has established tolerances and action levels for metals, such as for lead in a wide variety of grains and for mercury in certain kinds of wheat. Usually they enter the growing plant in the field, but occasionally toxic metals can also get into grains *after* harvest. I came across a couple of cases of lead contamination in stone-milled flour, which were caused by the lead joints used in the mills. Don't dismiss stone-milling as irrelevant to modern-day life. Stone-milled flour is readily available here—even for our homemade pizzas. My favorite local bakery makes stone-milled flour bread (with the flour fresh-milled every morning). I took a look at their mill just to make sure. The mill was beautiful, but mmmm, lead . . . another romantic notion destroyed! But still, in terms of probability, lead in your flour is a minor safety issue.

It looks as though arsenic in rice may turn out to be a more serious risk. As we know, arsenic is one of the worst heavy metals— literally a murder weapon. Children with pica, a disorder that makes them eat soil, can end up with toxic levels. It appears rice plants can absorb large quantities from arsenic-contaminated soil, although such grains as wheat and oats are likely to have lower arsenic levels. How much arsenic we are likely to get from our rice or rice products will be affected by the type that we eat, as well as where the rice has been grown. This is a relatively new issue, and the research findings are just emerging. There is still a great deal we don't know.

Studies have found frighteningly high amounts of arsenic, including of the more dangerous inorganic arsenic, in some rice crops grown by our trading partners such as India, Bangladesh, and China. In the United States, the levels of arsenic in rice will vary considerably between crops grown in one part of the country and those grown in another. In certain parts of the south-central United States, rice is grown on land where farmers previously grew cotton and used arsenic-based pesticides to control the boll weevils. Arsenic levels in such soil can be nearly twice as high as in Californian rice, and just as high as in certain Bangladeshi rice.

Organic growing conditions do not guarantee that rice will be low in arsenic. If the soil the rice grows in contains high levels, the arsenic will be soaked up by the rice plant, whether it is organically grown or inorganically grown. Wouldn't you know it, studies argue that brown rice—which has higher levels of bran and germ and is healthier for us—has higher levels of arsenic than does white rice. Rice bran will have much higher levels than both—ten to twenty times higher than in bulk rice grains. That is where the arsenic concentrates (see sidebar).

SUPERHEALTHY RICE BRAN WITH A TOUCH OF ARSENIC

Rice bran is now promoted as a healthy superfood. You can eat it or drink it. It turbo-charges your morning and winds you down at the end of the day. Years ago, it used to have a nasty cardboard taste. Now you can buy it in delicious chocolate, vanilla, and strawberry flavors.

Rice bran has been recognized by many health enthusiasts—and promoted by the industry—as a food people should eat if they have high cholesterol, poor digestion, or poor nutrition. That probably covers at least half the North American population. It has great vitamin and antioxidant content. It is gluten-free and a wonderful source of dietary fiber. It also contains rare enzymes, such as CoQ10, touted for strengthening the immune system, improving heart function, and even preventing cancer. These claims may be true—as long as these wonderful nutrients have not been destroyed during the rice bran–stabilizing process (heat treatment, with or without chemicals, to prevent spoilage).

Unfortunately there is a downside: this healthy food could give you too much arsenic, particularly for people who eat a lot of rice bran while also exposed to other sources of arsenic, or when rice bran solubles are used as a superfood, including for malnourished children in international aid programs. Too much arsenic could actually cause cancer—of the bladder, kidneys, skin, and other parts of the body. It can also lead to problems such as high blood pressure and loss of memory, which are not good, either—unless there are things we would rather forget.

"Safe" standards for arsenic intake are quite controversial. Continuous exposure to small amounts of arsenic can cause arsenic deposits in the body. But how much is too much? Arsenic is present in the drinking water of many countries, including the United Sates. We can be getting more than a little dose of arsenic every day of our lives. The EPA has set 10 ppb as the maximum level of arsenic allowed in U.S. drinking water. Presently, there are no standards for arsenic levels in our food, except for edible parts of animals that have been given arsenic-containing veterinary drugs (such as chickens and turkeys, discussed on page 149). Of course, we don't eat that much rice bran in a day but if we do get some arsenic from it, add some more from our drinking water, maybe some more from our beef (see page 170), a little from our rice grains, and a trace more from our lawn spray . . . so much for rice bran being a superhealthy food.

Limit Natural Toxins

Soybeans have sometimes been called "the king of beans." They are fast becoming the most important bean in the world. But certain research suggests that natural toxins, or "antinutrients," in soy may actually harm us if we get enough of them. Although other legumes and grains can also contain such toxic substances, soybeans are generally viewed as the riskiest. These toxins have occasionally been linked to such health problems as digestive disorders, immune system breakdown, thyroid dysfunction, diabetes, malnutrition, heart disease, infertility, precocious puberty, and even cancer. But the science behind such possible risks of eating soybeans and soy-based products is not conclusive (see sidebar). Our fears may turn out to be exaggerated.

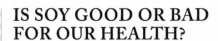

IS SOY GOOD OR BAD FOR OUR HEALTH?

Entire books have been written both on the wonderful health benefits of soy as well as on the antinutrients in soy. Which is correct? Is soy good or bad for us? The jury is still out.

Among the "negatives" often referred to are enzyme inhibitors that could prevent our body from properly digesting proteins, phytic acids—also present in bran and other legumes—that can reduce our absorption of certain essential minerals (such as magnesium, calcium, iron, and especially zinc), and a substance called hemagglutinin that causes red blood cells to clump together, potentially affecting proper absorption of oxygen. There are also isoflavones (a weak form of estrogen). Some studies I have looked at have shown a positive connection between isoflavones and the prevention and treatment of certain cancers, osteoporosis, and heart disease, as well as their providing relief for menopausal symptoms. However, other research has found a dangerous link between isoflavones and suppression of thyroid functioning, with special risks for infants on soy formula. Still other studies postulate a link between soy infant formula and changes in sexual development. As with many controversial food safety issues, other research—often quoted by the industry—appears to disprove such links. This is a very complex issue.

In addition to all these negative factors, a very high percentage of U.S.-grown soy is genetically modified—93 percent in 2010. Soy can also carry a heavy pesticide load.

Overall, eating small amounts of tofu is unlikely to cause us any harm. But if you want to keep eating soy and are a bit worried about these downside risks, eat it moderately and stick to what some experts argue to be the safer soy foods. These experts say that fermentation and cooking reduce at least some of the toxic risks although antinutrients will not be completely deactivated by cooking. In general, it is agreed that you would be safer eating fermented soy products such as miso and tempeh. Of course, never eat uncooked soybeans. Vegetarians who eat tofu and bean curd as a substitute for meat and dairy should check the latest research (including on how much soy is safe to consume). If your baby is allergic to cow's milk, read up on soy before switching to soy-based formula. There are many online sources. To avoid genetically modified soy and all those pesticides, eat organic.

Read Those Labels

Country of Origin Labeling (COOL)

As noted in earlier references to COOL (see page 77), this legislation only applies to the commodities that were specifically mentioned when it was passed. Grains were *not* mentioned, and are therefore not covered by the COOL requirements. Legumes are only partly covered. Fresh legumes would be, because they would meet the COOL definition of "perishable agricultural commodity." Processed or dry legumes are not. This means that retailers (most grocery stores and supermarkets) would have to provide country-of-origin information for fresh beans and sprouts but not for dried beans or lentils. In the case of peanuts, COOL legislation applies if they are raw but not if they are roasted, because roasting is defined as processing, and "processed food items" are excluded from COOL.

If you think the COOL requirements for grains and peanuts are odd, they are even more mysterious in the case of tree nuts. The USDA staff I consulted could not tell me why certain nuts are covered by COOL and others are not. The covered tree nuts are pecans and macadamia nuts. Other nuts such as almonds, cashews, pine nuts, and walnuts do not have to be labeled as to their country of origin. But in the end, even roasted pecans and macadamia nuts will be not be subject to COOL for the same reason roasted peanuts are not. But wait—if I understand the wording of the law correctly, then COOL would apply to raw macadamia nuts, but any chocolate-covered raw macadamia nuts would be excluded.

Organic Labeling

The term *organic* has the usual meaning when applied to grains, legumes, or nuts. All kinds of organic grains, legumes, and nuts are now available in the marketplace. In the case of a legume such as alfalfa, certified organic alfalfa sprout seed would need to be used. In the case of organic nuts, fumigants such PPO would not be allowed. Instead, they will probably have been subjected to a process such as steam sterilization.

Whole Grain

Whole-grain foods contain the entire grain, including germ, bran, and endosperm. Any food carrying the "whole grain" label has to meet FDA requirements for such labeling. Whole grains cover a wide range. The Whole Grains Council (a nonprofit consumer advocacy group working to increase consumption of whole grains for better health) provides a list of those most generally accepted in America (the ones in italics are not, strictly speaking "true grains" although used as such): *amaranth*, barley (lightly pearled), brown and colored rice, *buckwheat*, bulgur, corn and whole cornmeal, emmer, faro, grano (lightly pearled wheat), ramat grain, millet, oatmeal and whole oats, popcorn, *quinoa*, sorghum, spelt, triticale, whole rye, whole or cracked wheat, wheat berries, and wild rice. Even that is not a complete list. How many of these do you eat? There is a whole new world of grains out there.

The Whole Grains Council has also created a whole-grains packaging symbol—a stamp—to help consumers buy whole-grain products. It came out in 2005 and now appears on thousands of products and in many countries. There are actually two stamps: The "100%" stamp assures that a food contains a full serving or more of whole grain in each labeled serving and that *all* the grain is whole grain. The basic "whole grain" stamp appears on products containing at least *half* a serving of whole grain per labeled serving (see figure 9).

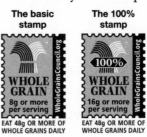

Figure 9

Raw Label on Nuts

The FDA permits both steam-treated and untreated almonds, cashews, and other nuts to be labeled "raw." Strictly speaking, the steam-sterilized nuts are not raw by raw-food-eater standards, as they have been heated to high temperatures. To obtain the truly raw ones will require going to a farmers' market or farm stand, preferably in California.

• • •

But What About . . . ?

Grain Questions

What is the safest rice to eat if I am afraid of arsenic?

Unfortunately, in terms of avoiding arsenic, available research points to white rice as probably being the safest—although it is the worst choice from a nutritional point of view (again—that frequent trade-off). Other than that, check where the rice is grown—that is, if you can find the information. Look for rice that is grown in such places as California, and avoid rice grown in certain sections of Kansas, where there is a lot of arsenic in the soil. Arsenic levels in imported rice also vary. At least some imported jasmine rice from Thailand and basmati rice from India have been found to contain low levels of arsenic—even less than most U.S.-grown rice.

Can arsenic contaminate baby foods made with rice?

It is possible. Fairly recently, researchers testing rice baby foods sold in UK supermarkets discovered that a large percentage of these products contained dangerously high levels of inorganic arsenic. I have not been able to locate any similar testing in North America. But there is no reason why it can't also happen here.

How can I avoid those dangerous mycotoxins in my corn cobs?

Fresh corn is usually considered a vegetable, but this question might as well be answered here. Dangerous mycotoxins in grains are produced only by certain molds, and even those do not produce them all the time. Unlike bacteria, fungi can usually—but not always—be seen. Peel back those corn husks in the store (and again, at home), and make sure that the cob does not have streaking or fuzzy areas. Buying local or organic will not protect you. I picked up some moldy organic local corn a couple of months ago.

Legume Questions

What should I look for to make sure peanuts in the shell are safe to eat?

Peanuts grown in the United States have to be certified as wholesome before they can be sold. But this does not mean that they can't become unhealthy later on. To be safe, check three things before you eat: that the peanut shells are unbroken, that the nuts don't rattle inside when you shake them, and that the peanuts are dry.

How can I tell if peanut butter is unsafe?

If peanut butter jars have legible code dates, you can use these as an indication of how long the product can be safely eaten. However, usually this is a conservative date and if the peanut butter has been properly stored (refrigerated), or not opened, it can be used a little longer. But if you open a jar of peanut butter and it smells rancid or has mold growth, throw it out.

Nut Questions

Which type of nuts are safest?

It is impossible to say which kind of nuts are safest. However, you can assume that, generally speaking, roasted nuts are safer to eat than raw nuts (yet again—raw is risky!), and nuts in shells are safer than shelled nuts. Shelling nuts decreases costs of transportation and storage, but it shortens their storage life and makes them more accessible to contaminants such as bacteria and mold, sometimes helped along by insects. If you plan to keep nuts for a long time, it is best to buy them in their shells, and store all nuts in the fridge.

What should I look for when buying tree nuts in shells?

When buying nuts in shells, use the same criteria as for peanuts. If you are buying them in open bins, take a quick sniff when no one is looking, to make sure they smell all right.

What should be done with nuts that taste bitter or if they have black spots?

If nuts taste bitter or rancid, or have black spots, holes, or other forms of discoloration, they are likely to be spoiled. While they may not always be unsafe, they should not be eaten. Besides, they usually taste awful.

Smart Ways to Reduce Your Risks

GROWING SAFE ALFALFA SPROUTS.

If you really insist on eating alfalfa or other sprouted seeds, then grow them yourself—but safely. The University of California–Davis, Division of Agriculture and Natural Resources, Publication #8151 has provided advice on how to adapt to small-scale home production the FDA safe-production guidance for commercial growers. I have never tried this, as I have stopped growing sprouts, so I offer no guarantees and have no idea if this affects growth, taste, or germination. The following summarizes the UC–Davis advice and adds a little extra safety from my side:

◇ Buy certified pathogen-free seed.

◇ Preheat a solution of 3 percent hydrogen peroxide (available at all drugstores) in a pot to 140°F. Immerse the seed in this solution for five minutes, maintaining a constant temperature and making sure that all the seed is heated uniformly. You could use something like a mesh strainer bag to hold the seed.

◇ Rinse the seed under running tap water for one minute.

◇ Pour out the hydrogen peroxide solution and put the rinsed seed back into the pot, covering it with clean, cold water and shaking lightly so that any debris floats to the top. Pour off or skim off this debris with a clean utensil and discard (most contaminants are likely to be there).

◇ Make sure you sanitize your sprouting containers before use with a bleach solution or similar, followed by multiple rinsings in cold water.

Buy the safest foods you can. With grains, legumes, and nuts, it is far less easy to tell what is fresh and what isn't than if you were buying fish or vegetables. One way to deal with this situation is simply to buy at a reliable store that has a fairly fast turnover. Be cautious with grains, peanuts, or nuts, sold in bulk, without labels, in small markets. Make sure that the nuts you buy are fresh (see page 262) and from a reputable company. If you are concerned about bacteria in your tree nuts (unlikely, but it can happen) then, much as you may be tempted, avoid buying raw nuts from roadside stands, unless you are sure they have been sterilized. You may also want to eat U.S.- or Canadian-grown and processed nuts or nut-derived products (most on the market *will* be domestic). But if pesticide residues are your concern and you still want to eat raw nuts, then make sure they have been steam-sterilized (or using another method that avoids PPO treatment). Or buy organic.

There is still a lot we don't know about the risks of longer-term exposure to heavy metals such as arsenic, but if it concerns you, be careful where your rice comes from (see page 258). This is more important if you tend to eat a lot of rice and may also be getting arsenic from other food or water sources. Also, be careful with superfood rice-bran products such as those found in health food stores and on the Internet. If you do want to consume such foods, do so in moderation and make sure you avoid arsenic from other sources.

Watch how you store foods. Once you have opened a vacuum-sealed package of nuts, refrigerate them in a sealed container. Shelled roasted nuts are likely to become rancid even sooner than fresh nuts, so don't assume that roasting will protect them. Also keep opened peanut butter and any other peanut-containing foods in the refrigerator. Keep an eye on the expiration or "best if used by" date. Keep grains, legumes, and nuts dry, as well as crackers and snacks made from grains or legumes. If they look or feel limp, throw them out. Also keep your grain cereals and grain-based foods dry, particularly when the kitchen environment is warm.

Wash. It is always wise to rinse uncooked rice and dried beans, lentils, and other legumes, and throw out any debris that rises to the surface. Ever since I broke a tooth on a small stone that looked like a lentil, I always check for them by sorting the lentils on a large plate. Although a boring task, it is cheaper and less time-consuming than fixing a broken tooth. Washing raw sprouts may help a bit, but is not likely to remove any bacteria that have got inside the seed—which is the usual pattern. In other words, don't rely on it. Don't wash nuts, unless you want to do it right before using them in a cooked dish.

Cook well. Make sure that all baked goods, including savory items such as meat or chicken pies, are thoroughly cooked before you eat them, particularly if you are using a microwave. One way to make your alfalfa safer, too, is to cook it, as the government gurus advise. But who wants to eat cooked alfalfa?

Watch what you eat. Never eat raw cookie dough; nuts that taste bitter, odd, or are no longer crunchy; and any grain or grain-based foods, such as bread, tortillas, or burritos, that have developed mold (I hate to admit it, but my quinoa bread frequently reaches that point when I forget about it). Wash your hands well after making cookies, or if you have touched moldy breads, odd-looking nuts, or even raw sprouted seeds. Only eat commercially sold raw sprouts if you want a change from gambling on the stock market, and want to do it with your health instead.

Diversify. Diversification is a particularly useful safety rule for grains. In other words, it is a good idea not to consume a large helping of rice or corn tortillas three times a day, or eat eight cups of rice or massive quantities of soy foods. Yes, this may be done in some countries—where people tend to have much shorter life spans than we hope for. Instead, you may want to try some of the wonderful whole-grain alternatives that are now being sold more widely in the United States, such as quinoa.

Be extra careful when eating out. Read the menu carefully, and ask for raw sprouts not to be put on your sandwiches and salads. (Sometimes, when I have forgotten, I have pulled them off afterward, but they may already have contaminated the lettuce or tomato underneath.) At banquets and large catered affairs, you may want to think twice before eating those wonderful-looking cakes and desserts—not just for protecting your waistline and cholesterol, but also to avoid contaminants such as norovirus. If you want an incentive not to order dessert next time you eat out, remember my true story of the "instant" chocolate birthday cake.

10

Herbs and Spices

Are spices dangerous? Yes, that tiny pinch of pepper or just a few basil leaves can carry enough contaminants to hurt you. Even the dried ones. As a devoted herb and spice user (I think there are around one hundred herb and spice containers in my kitchen), I find that particularly annoying.

However, in general, herbs and spices figure less frequently in outbreaks of food-borne illnesses. They also result in fewer incidents of illness than do produce, fish, dairy, eggs, meat, or poultry. But it is quite likely that they are the last suspect, even if they are guilty of making us sick. It could also be that herbs and spices are at least partly responsible for some of our longer-term problems.

What We Use

American and Canadian consumers, restaurants, and food processing companies have begun to use more and more herbs and spices over the years. Herbs and spices not only make our food taste better but they can also help preserve it and reduce the amount of unhealthy salt we use. Between 1980 and 2000, our annual consumption of spices more than doubled, and it is still increasing. We only consume about half of those spices in home cooking. The other half goes to the food industry and food-service sector.

Did you know that much of that great taste in such processed foods and beverages as meat products, gravy mixes, salad dressings, soups, baked goods—and even in soft drinks and candy—is due to the spice ingredients? Even fast-food chains are major herb and spice users. Any fast food hamburger, fried chicken, or pizza is likely to carry a few, such as pepper, paprika, oregano, and more. Spices are also frequently used in ready-to-eat foods, including deli products. Remember how boring the sliced turkey used to taste before it was coated with pepper? And what do you think is in that pepperoni?

Another reason we eat herbs and spices—apart from taste—is that we think some of them are good for us: They could improve our digestion, boost our immune system, lower our blood pressure and cholesterol, reduce inflammation, give us energy, help us sleep better, and reduce our risk of cancer. In fact, in many countries, herbs and certain spices have been in use for medical purposes for centuries. Several have long been believed to actually kill microbes. I was brought up with such beliefs: "Always drink chamomile tea at bedtime." "Turmeric is good for arthritis." "If you think you are getting a cold, take a dose of chili pepper." "Take garlic pills to protect you against parasites."

Perhaps before going further, it would be a good idea to sort out the difference between herbs and spices. They are often referred to together, as we are also doing here, but they are actually quite different:

- **Spices** generally come from the root, seeds, bark, flowers, or fruit of a plant.
- **Herbs** are derived from the green part (leaves or stem) of plants that do not have a woody stem.

There are a few exceptions to this rule. One is rosemary, which we view as an herb for cooking purposes, but is really a shrub. Herbs are often used in fresh form as well as dried. A few, such as cilantro and coriander, are both herb and spice respectively, from the same plant.

Let's look at spices first. Among the more commonly used spices in North America are chili pepper, cinnamon, cloves, cumin, ginger, mustard, nutmeg, paprika, pepper (black and white), vanilla bean, and the spice blend known as curry (actually a mixture of spices such as turmeric, cumin, and coriander; there are many variations of curry powder ingredients and proportions). Some spices such as annatto seed, paprika, saffron, and turmeric are used to give color as well as flavor.

Over half of our spices that we use in North America are imported. Spice imports have grown rapidly. They originate in maybe as many as one hundred warmer foreign countries—places such as Indonesia, Mexico, India, Egypt, and China. By weight, China is now the leading country of origin for spices to the United States. In all, we import about forty different spices. Those we import in greatest quantity are capsicums, cinnamon, mustard seeds, pepper (black and white), sesame seed, and vanilla beans. Such spices tend to arrive at our ports in large sacks or paper bags, are subjected to fumigation or other methods of sterilization, and cleaned or reconditioned, if need be. The half or so that goes to retailers or industrial settings arrives in large, sealed containers. We get ours in the store or online in small tins, jars, or packages. The United States is now the largest spice importer and consumer in the world.

Many of the herbs we eat, however, can be grown in our own backyard, on a sunny patio, or even in our kitchen. That is, if we don't forget to water them (I often do). Among our favorite herbs are basil, chives, cilantro, dill, marjoram, mint, oregano, parsley, rosemary, sage, sesame seeds, thyme, and tarragon. A longer and more complete list of herbs and spices in common use is provided by the American Spice Trade Association (ASTA) on their Web site. ASTA also includes as spices two bulb vegetables, considered "aromatics" rather than herbs or spices, which are sometimes sold in dehydrated form: garlic and onion. China is also our biggest source of garlic.

Who Keeps It Safe?

IN THE UNITED States, the FDA is responsible for ensuring that spices are not adulterated or misbranded. It inspects and samples imported spice shipments as well as domestically grown ones to check for organisms or anything else that could harm us—such as unapproved additives or colorings or other substances that should not be there. The FDA also tries to make sure that no unknown or unapproved spices are entering our markets.

The spice industry organizations, like ASTA, play a key role in safety as well. Founded in 1907, ASTA represents most of the companies that grow, dehydrate, and process spices in the United States as well as U.S.-based spice agents, brokers, and importers, and overseas companies that grow and ship spices to America. If you look at ASTA activities and its history, you will notice its active involvement in formulating safety regulations—as do some other industry bodies we have mentioned. An example is the ASTA Cleanliness Specifications for Unprocessed Spices, Seeds and Herbs, developed in 1969 and revised twelve times since, in consultation with its membership (no government agency keeps guidelines that well updated). ASTA also informs its members of any proposed new safety measures (such as for disinfection, storage, or handling), and, if mandated, encourages and educates members about how to apply them in their own activities.

The spice industry is complex and changing. Although the domestic market is dominated by a few large companies (such as McCormick), it is believed that in the United States there are close to ten thousand consignees that buy imported spices. And there are hundreds of spice manufacturers in countries such as

India, China, and Mexico, which are sending us their products. Goodness only knows how many thousands of smaller spice producers they rely on, or what, if any, oversight these receive. I try not to think about some of the practices I have seen farmers and processors using in the countries in which I have worked. Some foreign growers and processors and some domestically based importers are very safety conscious and responsible. Others simply don't know better or hope they won't get caught.

Bacteria-Poisoned Pepper

THE LARGE MAJORITY of spices eaten in the United States can be considered fairly safe from bacteria. The reason is that 70 to 80 percent of those that are imported, and even domestically traded ones, will be sold under an ASTA contract. This contract requires high standards of cleanliness. In addition, every single shipment of spices is tested in accredited laboratories. (Compare this with USDA testing of 2 to 4 percent testing of spices.) If it fails, then it is given one second chance to be "reconditioned" (see page 269) and retested. Or it is sent back. Of course, there are still the difficulties of sampling of large shipments of spices, making it vital to collect samples throughout the whole (see discussion with regard to grains, page 238). There is also the fact that the very large majority of bacteria will not be tested for. Even so, the vigilance of ASTA, plus several of its other activities, such as spice supplier education (including overseas) certainly helps. This would argue that the spices that are most likely to carry contaminants, including bacteria, are the other 20 or so percent that are not processed through ASTA. The companies involved are likely to be the smaller ones.

You might be surprised at how many cases of contamination of herbs and spices, including dried ones, do continue to occur. In fact, spice-related outbreaks have increased, but this could have something to do with our using more of them. During one 2009 six-month period I looked at, twelve recalls were announced—

four for herbs and eight for spices. Outbreaks have been most often associated with those spices and dried herbs we commonly use—such as different kinds of pepper and parsley, cilantro, and basil. But *any* herb or spice can carry bacteria.

In dried spices and herbs, most of the culprit bacteria involved have been one or other of the *Salmonella* genus, which are proving that they don't mind such dry (or spicy) conditions. And, as we have found out, these days these bacteria are everywhere in our food. In fact, all eight cases of spice contamination during that six-month period in 2009 were caused by one or other *Salmonella* bacterium. Most outbreaks were multistate and many involved different kinds of spices. I counted twenty-five different spices with *Salmonella* problems in just one year alone—even involving the hottest spice. Research has shown that *Salmonella* can survive in cayenne pepper for months.

The very large majority of *spice* contaminations have involved imported spices, which is not surprising in view of the fact that most of our spices come from overseas. I took a look at the FDA's rejection of herb and spice import shipments by country during the last four years. At least fifteen shipments from Egypt were found to contain *Salmonella* bacteria, including ones of sweet basil, bay leaves, dill, whole and ground cumin, fennel, mint, sweet marjoram, oregano, and sesame seed and paste. During the same period, FDA inspectors also stopped at least twelve *Salmonella*-contaminated shipments of spices and dried herbs from China, including shipments of anise, cayenne pepper, celery seed, five-spice powder, mixed spice, black peppercorns, and sesame seed, as well as ginger in whole, cracked, and powdered form.

The bacteria situation in *fresh herbs* is more varied. Although *Salmonella* are still commonly involved in outbreaks, in several cases the culprit has been the toxin-producing *E. coli*. But *Salmonella* in parsley and/or cilantro—just these two herbs alone—has been causing at least one or two outbreaks every year. In instances, as many as five hundred illnesses have been reported. Some of the herbs involved have been grown overseas, in countries such as Mexico.

The labels on others have implied that they were grown in the United States. But we consumers are now aware that a product with a label such as "California Naturally Healthy Herbs" (a fictitious name) does not guarantee that it was grown in California. It could originate in the Mexicali Valley, produced under contract to U.S. growers. That is cheaper for the industry. But is it as safe for us?

How do herbs and spices become contaminated? As with other plants, they come into contact with soil, dust, and water, as well as fecal material from birds, rats, and roaming animals. It's picturesque to see red chili peppers being dried along the side of a road, but the reality is less romantic. A lot of spices are dried in the sun—and amid the dust and fumes of passing traffic. Again, as always, spices may be exposed to contaminated equipment, contaminated water (as when peppercorns are soaked to prepare white pepper), or plant workers who carry microbes (sometimes showing no symptoms).

Yes, drying of spices normally reduces the numbers of bacteria. But it will not completely eliminate them. The food industry uses methods such as irradiation (see pages 71 and 158), steam, and fumigants to make spices safer. The main fumigant used on spices in the United States is not approved in many other countries (see page 276). There is no guarantee that all our spices have received such treatment, particularly those that do not enter the country under ASTA regulations. There are so many dealers in spices in North America. Nor is there any guarantee that they will not become contaminated *after* such treatment.

POISONED PEPPER

In spring 2009, the FDA was informed that several people who had eaten Asian restaurant food in Portland, Oregon, had become ill. When that happens, the first assumption would be to suspect bad hygiene or poor food preparation practices at the restaurant. But the people who became ill had not gone to the same restaurant; they had dined at several different ones. This changed the picture. As it was unlikely the establishments passed the chicken chow mein or fried rice back and forth, it pointed to some food product or ingredient they all bought (such as fortune cookies), or some cooking ingredient they all used.

An investigation was launched that eventually involved the FDA, the CDC, and state health officials in California, Oregon, Nevada, and Washington. It was discovered that what was making everyone ill was a rare *Salmonella rissen* bacterium. This bacterium finally turned up at the restaurants in an unexpected place—in the pepper containers kept on the tables so that customers could sprinkle it onto their food if it lacked pizzazz. The pepper—imported from China—had been packed and distributed to these restaurants by a California-based food company, Union International Food Co. It turned out that the contaminated products had been sold—under different brand names—to several Asian supermarkets, distributors, and wholesalers, as well as to (mostly Chinese) restaurants.

As usually happens in cases of food contamination these days, especially if a food ingredient is involved, the outbreak turned out to be much bigger than initially suspected. In the end, it extended to five states. The confirmed illness count was close to eighty people in California, Nevada, Oregon, Washington, and Idaho. Investigators found that the illnesses had actually begun about six months earlier. (These recalls and alerts usually get off to a slow start.) In the end, the company responsible had to recall several of its peppers (black, white, and cayenne); plus curry powder, garlic, chopped dried onion and onion powder, and wasabi powder; as well some sauces, oils, and oil blends in various size packages.

You may want to think twice before you lift up that pepper shaker in a restaurant next time. Maybe you can live without it.

The FDA considers spices to be ready-to-eat products—that is, foods that are prepared in advance and can be safely eaten without any additional washing or cooking. We also tend to assume that they don't need a "kill" step. But it might be a good idea to do it anyway, particularly if you are in a high-risk group. Rather than sprinkle spices like chili pepper or black or white pepper onto your food before you eat it—cook it into the food.

Parasites in Fresh Herbs?

HERBS SUCH AS black walnut, garlic, goldenseal, and wormwood have been used for centuries to help avoid or to treat intestinal parasites. But parasites can also contaminate herbs. It usually happens while they are growing in the field. Feces-contaminated irrigation water is frequently the cause, as it is with produce. Rosemary and tarragon are probably the safest from parasites because they grow higher off the ground. Other fresh herbs such as basil, cilantro, parsley, and basil can easily become contaminated. Because we often eat them raw, such parasites can be alive and well when the herbs enter our mouth. Not a pleasant thought. But at present they do not seem to be as much of a risk as are bacteria. This could change. As mentioned before, microbes are evolving all the time, and our global food supply brings with it new risks.

THERE COULD BE *CYCLOSPORA* IN YOUR BASIL

Cyclospora (see page 58) is a "coccidian parasite that causes outbreaks of protracted and relapsing **gastroenteritis**." In plain English, that means that it is a nasty small protozoa that can give you on-and-off diarrhea, fever, chills, and other unpleasant symptoms for a long time. *Cyclospora cayetanensis* is quite common in such countries as Peru, Egypt, and Nepal, and was first identified in humans in Papua New Guinea. That makes it a nicely traveled global problem.

Over the years in the United States and Canada, *Cyclospora* has been associated with several outbreaks involving fresh basil, including organic basil (as well as mesclun mixes, raspberries, and snow peas—see page 59). In fact, out of the twenty-four *Cyclospora* outbreaks listed in the database of the Center for Science in the Public

Interest (CSPI), three, or possibly four, traced back to basil. In some cases, its presence in basil has caused close to six hundred illnesses. This is quite impressive, given that only a small percentage of people eat fresh basil in the first place.

Again, Toxic Molds

SPICES CAN ALSO become contaminated with molds, as can many of our foods. Some of these molds can harm our health if they produce high levels of aflatoxin or other mycotoxins (see page 54). Some of the spices that have been found to carry such mold toxins have included cardamom, cinnamon, clove, coriander, cumin, ginger, and black pepper, and red chili pepper. (However, some research I founds suggests that cinnamon and clove, along with oregano and thyme, may actually be quite resistant to such molds). Mold growth and toxin production will be influenced by temperature, humidity, and even the type of packing materials used for the spices. As always, in North America the main risk is low-level long-term exposure, not a large dose in a single meal.

Another Pesticide Issue

THE SPICE INDUSTRY regularly uses toxic fumigants. This helps to prevent contamination of spices by those nasty bacteria such as *Salmonella* and *E. coli*. It also prevents introduction of new agricultural pests through the imported spices or their packaging materials. True, we do not want deadly bacteria or agricultural contaminants in our spices, but we don't want unhealthy pesticide residues, either. It is the same dilemma as in the case of fumigation of nuts (see previous chapter). And it prompts yet again the same question: Is the trade-off worth it?

More than half of our spices—and maybe as much as 85 percent—are treated with the fumigant ethylene oxide (EtO).

This chemical is used primarily to sterilize medical equipment. Other alternatives for treating our spices *are* available, such as irradiation, steam sterilization, or exposure to ozone or carbon dioxide. But the industry prefers fumigation, as some of these alternatives do not work as well on both insects *and* bacteria, or may affect the appearance or flavor of the spices. (Remember, the nut industry likes the fumigant PPO for the same reasons). But what about the residues EtO leaves in the spices? And what about the fact that the IARC has reclassified EtO as a known human carcinogen? And what about the fact that many other countries have banned the use of EtO as a fumigant for foods or spices, due to such health concerns about the residues it leaves?

What seems clear is that the FDA *has been* worried—and maybe still is. When EtO came up for reregistration in 2006–2008, the agency gave the industry trade organization ASTA a choice: Either prove that ethylene chlorohydrin (ECH)—a possible residue from EtO use—is not carcinogenic, or reduce the level of these residues in spices. ASTA was able to do the latter by developing different procedures for application of EtO (only basil could not meet those new standards). Note the key role that ASTA has played in this. But is there still risk?

ASTA's own research showed that the earlier levels of residues left in spices by EtO *were* way, way too high, especially for infants and children. For instance, in children one to two years of age, it was 650 percent of the population-adjusted dose (PAD) now considered acceptable, and for three- to twelve-year-olds it was 580 percent of it. Remember—the changed tolerances only took effect in September 2009—after years of poorly regulated EtO use (the industry was given about two years to adjust to the new procedures). Some North American children consume from an early age quite a lot of EtO-sprayed herbs and spices in soft drinks, pizza, and fast foods. Even with improved treatment methods, the levels for children less than five years old barely meet the new safety requirements. That is, assuming the industry members actually comply with these new and safer residue limits. As I understand it, there is no requirement to *test* spices for EtO or ECH residues.

The EPA's decision to approve the use of EtO also came with a qualification—it would do further study of the longer-term carcinogenic effects of this fumigant. If such further study strengthens the case for risks, the EPA could change its mind—as it does all the time.

At this point, the research is still not perfectly clear on possible links between small amounts of EtO residues in our spices and longer-term health effects. One argument, which has been made by the WHO, is that such residues are unlikely to do us any harm, because they disappear over time. There does not appear to be complete agreement on this. Of course, there is an alternative: organic herbs and spices are readily available. Their growers and manufacturers use neither synthetic pesticides nor irradiation, and instead tend to rely on steam sterilization (see page 282). In fact, some not-for-profits are now encouraging small farmers in developing countries to grow herbs and spices for the North American markets, using their traditional farming techniques and know-how for composting, crop rotation, and biological control of pests and plant disease.

To tell the truth, I have been rather impressed with ASTA—probably more than with any other food industry organization (that is, if we define spices as a "food"). Its transparency is a factor. So I feel the need to balance the picture in terms of ASTA's role in pesticide use. ASTA *does* encourage its overseas suppliers, where possible, to use **integrated pest management (IPM)**—which is a fascinating, low-input approach to pest control. If they *must* use pesticides, ASTA encourages them to follow U.S. regulations. But I wonder how often this is being done. I took a look at these new procedures for EtO use and found them to be very precise. Perhaps I have just seen too much incorrect use of pesticides by farmers and farmworkers in developing countries—often simply because they were illiterate or semiliterate, and unable to read and follow instructions.

Can There Be Lead in Our Spices?

AT PRESENT, LEAD, arsenic, and such other heavy metals do not appear to be a big risk in our herbs and spices. However, some research both in the U.S. and Canada suggests that certain spices *may* have low levels. Could this have any connection to the fact that as many as one out of six U.S. children has frighteningly high blood levels of lead—with no known lead-paint cause for about a third of them? So how did it happen? It is speculated that some of the possible sources could be lead in soil, in ceramic dishes, lead in children's jewelry and toys—*and,* lead in their food. Food and such other nonpaint sources of lead risk are not well studied. We may have underestimated them.

Although food is a comparatively minor factor, it can add to what children—and adults—acquire from other sources. Foods that are known to sometimes be contaminated with lead are chocolate (as a chocoholic, I try not to think about this) and certain spices, such as chili pepper, curry powder, paprika, turmeric, and foods made with such spices. Lead poisoning is of greatest risk to infants, children, and pregnant women. In children, it could be contributing to common behavior problems and learning difficulties.

Lead could enter spices at almost any point during processing, from heavy lead-contamination of the soil, pots or tools used in grinding, contact with fine paint fragments in dust (as when spices are dried by the side of a busy road), or even packaging. Lead can also enter from any lead-contaminated water used in washing of spices.

Large doses of lead can be fatal. Two often-quoted incidents of severe lead poisoning in America involved two family groups that bought spices on overseas trips (one traveling to India, the other to Georgia). They then used these spices to cook meals back in America—and became seriously ill. The children in the families were particularly badly affected and had to be hospitalized. Such acute poisoning incidents from food are believed to be very rare in North America.

But cases *have* been reported in such places as Boston and various parts of California, of chronic lead poisoning due to the ingestion of cultural powders or spices (from India, Nepal, Bangladesh—not sold in large stores). Chili pepper may have been the culprit in dangerously high levels of lead that were discovered in 2009 in several brands and types of spicy imported candy and chewing gum. Lead-contaminated chili powder had also been suspected in earlier candy recalls, in 2004 and 2007. Much of this contaminated candy originated in Mexico, and some in Malaysia. Obviously lead-laced candy is particularly bad because most children eat candy.

Small studies have compared lead levels in known-brand spices distributed by the larger spice companies with those sold in small packages in certain specialty-stores. The latter were found to frequently have higher lead levels. But this does not mean that some small companies are not safe—or even safest. Some of the best organic companies routinely test for heavy metals in all their herbs and spices and discard any that do not meet safety standards. Still, it does suggest that we should be careful in buying unknown label spices. Spices that we use at home or in our processed foods (including . . . sigh . . . chocolate) could be gradually building up too much lead in our body.

DANGEROUS DYES ARE UNLIKELY

As far as we know, dangerous dyes in spices are a very minor risk in North America. But, it could happen. Some are being caught by spice inspections at our borders. As we now know, if inspection catches some, it means that more are getting through—although less likely with those under ASTA contract.

Usually one or other of the "Sudan dyes" is involved in any problems. The IARC has classified several Sudan dyes as category 3 carcinogens, a classification used when the experts are not ready to commit themselves, but are worried. Such dyes are perfectly fine for coloring waxes and shoe polish. But you want them in your ketchup or your pasta?

The United States and Canada do not allow the use of Sudan dyes and similar toxic synthetic dyes in foods and spices. However, some of the countries from which we import spices are still using such dyes for intensifying the color of chili powder, curry powder, paprika, and other products. Obviously, an attractively colored spice fetches a better price, and these dyes are cheap to use. If they do get into the country, they could end up in foods such as tomato sauces, virgin palm oil, Worcestershire sauce, and even sausage products that are made with these spice ingredients. There have been a few recorded instances where this has actually happened, or the incoming products have been turned back at our ports. In recent years, FDA inspectors have also caught vanilla products coming in from the Philippines, Mexico, Dominican Republic, and Haiti to contain the banned FD&C Red #2 dyes. But overall, toxic dyes in spices seem to be less of a problem than some of our other risks.

Read Those Labels

LABELS ON OUR herbs or spices are of little help in helping us to be safe.

Country-of-Origin Labeling (COOL)

Dried herbs and spices were not covered by COOL requirements when the legislation was passed. However, fresh herbs, such as fresh basil, cilantro, mint, parsley, tarragon, thyme, and others, would classify under "perishable agricultural commodity" and have to comply with COOL (see page 77).

Natural Flavoring or Natural Spices

The FDA defines a "natural" flavor or flavoring as, "the essential oil, oleoresin, essence or extractive, protein hydrolysate, distillate, or any product of roasting, heating or enzymolysis, which contains the flavoring constituents derived from a spice, fruit or fruit juice, vegetable or vegetable juice, edible yeast, herb, bark, bud, root, leaf or similar plant material, meat, seafood, poultry, eggs, dairy products, or fermentation products thereof, whose significant function in food is flavoring rather than nutritional." According to this definition, spices are a "natural" flavoring. Therefore, to say that a spice is a "natural" spice is a statement of the obvious. If a spice is not "natural," it is not a spice. And to be labeled "natural" is by no means the same as being certifiably "organic." Therefore, this label has no safety implications. It may have even less in the future. USDA is working on changing the definition of the term *natural*.

On behalf of its members, ASTA has petitioned that the definition be allowed to include EtO-treated spices. The decision is pending at the present time.

Organic

Certified organic spices need to conform to the usual standards of organic production, as outlined in earlier chapters. Such production of herbs and spices tries to rely on biological forms of pest management, composting, and other similar techniques to increase yields and protect the crop from pests. Postharvest, organic spices are not allowed to be treated with fumigants such as EtO or with irradiation. Other techniques such as steam sterilization are employed to reduce bacteria levels and for killing insects and their eggs. Some of the better organic herb and spice companies also conduct a comprehensive testing of their products for bacteria, mold, heavy metals, and other possible contaminants before releasing them into the marketplace. In some instances, they are also much fresher than those sold by the larger companies, but this is not a requirement.

. . .

But What About . . . ?

Can insects invade herbs and spices?

Yes, they can. Sometimes the eggs are present in the original herb or spice, which was not irradiated, and then hatch in your kitchen. These insects are not necessarily dangerous in themselves, although they could carry bacteria or mold spores. And who wants to cook a pasta sauce containing wormy basil? Throw it out—before the insects spread in your kitchen.

Are dried or powdered chilis too unsafe to use?

True, dried or powdered chilis have been involved in several *Salmonella*-related recalls in recent years. There is also a remote possibility that this spice could contain one of the banned Sudan dyes (see page 280). But during some periods of time (1970–2003), paprika has been even more frequently contaminated. In comparison to some other food products we eat, the chances of finding pathogenic bacteria in your dried spices are relatively small. However, if you are worried, cook the powder or the chili seeds within the dish—don't sprinkle them over the food afterward. If you want to be more certain that brightly colored spices have not been colored with dangerous *dyes*, buy from a reputable company.

Is prepeeled fresh garlic as safe as whole cloves of garlic?

No. They are convenient, but peeled cloves are *less* safe. I hate peeling garlic, so I am always very tempted to buy them. At the same time, I know that the peeling process can introduce contaminants, as with any such processing step. The exposed tissues of the garlic cloves will also allow easier entry. At the time when I was still buying such peeled cloves, I bought a container from my favorite retailer, only to arrive back home and notice that several were covered with white mold. Of course, the retailer blamed their new supplier, but they should also have regularly checked the contents of their refrigerated display cabinet. And true, I was careless, too. Bottom line: People in high-risk groups should buy whole garlic cloves or use sterilized garlic flakes or powder.

Is it dangerous to use spices such as pepper when eating out?

Yes, it may be a bit risky, especially in the cheaper restaurants. You have no way of knowing the source of the pepper or other spice, how old it is, or how it has been stored. Just assume that many restaurants try to cut costs and buy the cheapest, particularly during an economic downturn. If you have a compromised immune system and know you will want to add spices when eating out, take along a pinch from home in your pocket—in a sealed bag, of course. That's what you call really planning ahead!

Smart Ways to Reduce Your Risks

WITH HERBS AND spices, as with foods in general, "raw" and "remote" can increase the risk. But we now know that even the most innocent-looking dried and processed spice may not be so innocent at all. Unfortunately, most of our seasonings are "remote." They come from distant and warmer countries. Even though many items are classified as "ready-to-eat," it would be wiser to assume that they are safer cooked. As for fresh herbs, local or home-grown organic is generally likely to be safest.

Grow your own herbs. Growing your own herbs is certainly the best way to ensure that they are as safe as possible. And just think of all the things you can do with just one plant of rosemary. You can use it in food preparation, potpourri, homemade astringent cosmetics, as a hair lotion to lighten the color and prevent baldness, as an insect repellant and disinfectant, for putting in a wedding wreath (or handing out at funerals—as in Wales), and to give to your lover as an ancient emblem of fidelity. But remember that those insects and birds flying around (and your cat or dog or that pesky raccoon) can even contaminate your home-garden herbs, so protect and clean them accordingly. You may also want to try growing pots of herbs in your kitchen on a sunny counter, on a patio, or even hang them from the ceiling, which can look very attractive (though watering is complicated).

Buy carefully. Even if you grow some herbs, you are still likely to have to buy the occasional bunch (particularly if the birds ate your basil, as in my case). In North America, you will also have to buy your spices. I have to admit that I used to buy any old herb or spice, and generally like to support small and local companies. But now I realize that I have to be a smarter buyer. That applies especially to basil, paprika, and black, white, and chili peppers, Your risks are likely to be lower if you buy dried herbs and spices in closed containers (jars, tins) distributed by a reputable company. In the case of fresh herbs, buy them locally grown and organic (in person from the actual farmer, if you can, so you can ask how they were grown) and avoid those that could be imported from countries where the irrigation water is frequently contaminated (in spite of COOL, fresh herbs seem to rarely be labeled. So I ask). There is no proof that irradiated spices are bad for us. But buy organic if you want to avoid pesticides and irradiation.

Store your herbs and spices correctly. Store your *fresh* commercially sold herbs, fresh turmeric or ginger root, curry leaves, and poppy seeds in the refrigerator, in the fruit and vegetable section. Keep them in their original wrapping, or loosely wrap them in plastic. If you have a lot in your garden or have bought in bulk, you may want to dry or freeze some for future use (There are good instructions on the Internet on how to do this). Sometimes when I pick herbs from my own garden such as basil, cilantro, mint, parsley, or rosemary, and I plan to use them in a day or so, I simply arrange them like flowers in a vase—a scented arrangement. But you need to change the water daily, and they won't keep well for more than a few days, unless placed in the fridge. Keep your *dried* herbs and spices in a dry, cool place, in sealed containers (not next to the stove, or in the refrigerator). Throw out any that are clumping together, look odd, or are old, to avoid bacteria and mold toxins. You may simply want to shake the container or rub some between your fingers, to make sure the herb or spice still has a scent; elderly herbs smell like hay and have little flavor, even if they are safe to use.

How long you keep herbs or spices has a lot to do with quality as well as safety. Spices, and especially dried herbs, tend to lose their strength as they age. Many seasonings have use-by dates on them these days. Ideal storage times will vary. It depends on what condition you bought them in. It also has to do with the type of herb or spice. Some whole spices, such as cinnamon sticks, whole cloves, nutmeg, and peppercorns, can be kept for ages if stored properly. Although opinions vary, you may want to generally think of the following time frames, even though there are exceptions of people surviving after eating forty-year-old spices in their Thanksgiving dinner.

- **Fresh herbs:** 3 to 7 days (in the refrigerator, longer if frozen)
- **Dried herbs:** 1 to 3 years
- **Ginger root, turmeric root:** up to a month (in the refrigerator, longer if frozen)
- **Ground spices:** 2 to 3 years
- **Whole spices:** up to 4 years

Use only herbs and spices meant for culinary use. Never cook or bake with dried or "stovetop" potpourri ingredients, fresh flower buds or petals that came from a florist's shop, or essential oils not specifically labeled as safe to consume, as they could make you very ill.

Wash your herbs. Yes, fresh herbs need to be washed well, preferably with three rinses of clean water, even though some of them will look pretty miserable by the time you are through. Even wash your rosemary, unless you are collecting it straight after a heavy rainstorm, as I did just now. Spin dry in a salad spinner, or blot well before using. There is no need to wash spices.

Cook when you can. Remember that as always, cooking your spices or your herbs is a type of "kill" step for bacteria or parasites that could be present.

Don't give your young children too many spices. It could be that fumigant residues in spices will not harm your child. But you may want to be careful, particularly with children under twelve years of age. When making food that they will also share, you may want to buy organic herbs and organic spices, which have been sterilized using alternative approaches.

When eating out, take it easy on the pepper shaker. That is, avoid sprinkling dried chili pepper, paprika, or other pepper or mixed spices onto your food after it has been brought to your table. It is also a good idea to remember that certain fast foods, or Asian or Mexican dishes that you may be ordering for your children, contain a lot of spices.

Take care when introducing new herbs and herbal products to your kitchen. Many traditional herbs are perfectly safe, but remember that just because they are natural doesn't mean all are safe to eat . . . or even touch. This includes many commonly availably herbal supplements, teas, ethnic products, and "old wives' tale" remedies. Lovage, to take just one example, can add a delightful celery-like flavor to dishes, but should be avoided by pregnant women because it is an abortifacient. If in doubt, consult an herb guide or a handbook of poisonous plants before using herbs with which you are not familiar.

Don't buy spices on overseas trips to bring back with you.
Except perhaps from EU countries. (I am trying to forget about
that time I bought saffron in the market in Marrakesh to bring
back home.)

Enjoy. Herbs and spices help us prepare delicious meals—particularly
if you have grown those herbs yourself.

11

No Final Word

There is no such thing as a final word on food safety. Our food system is changing. Food risks are changing. We are changing. The moment we think that something can't happen, it will. The moment we think that *we* can never get ill from our food, we will.

I recently spoke to a friend I hadn't seen for a few days. When I started to write this book, she told me that she had never had any problems with her food. Now, when I asked her how she had been, she said, "I have been really sick. We both [she and her husband] have been. A bad case of stomach flu . . ."

"You mean food poisoning?"

"No—stomach flu," she said. "Somehow or other we caught it when we went south to that wedding I told you about. The doctor put us on antibiotics . . ."

I didn't argue the point. Food poisoning is often mistaken for so-called stomach flu.

Risky food is everywhere.

And you can never predict what will be the next tainted food. I have just closed my overloaded e-mail inbox. Part of the load was due to alerts from the FDA and USDA. Unless I missed some, just in the last five days alone these two agencies have announced six sizeable food product recalls (not counting those for mislabeling or undeclared allergens, or for contaminated pet food). This is not an atypical number. Today's recall is for RTE bagged sliced apples, believed to be contaminated by *Listeria monocytogenes* bacteria. A few days ago there was one for RTE avocado pulp, also with *Listeria monocytogenes* suspected. Still another was for fresh peppers in which *Salmonella* may be hiding. And here is a recall for RTE bagged fresh spinach, this time with *E. coli* O157:H7 involved. There was also one announced for fully cooked RTE turkey breast (*L. monocytogenes*), plus a recall for ground bison meat (fresh), again with *E. coli* O157:H7 suspected. Most of these recalls are large, involving multiple U.S. states. In several cases, I suspect that we have already eaten much of the foods. There are, of course, many more than six products involved since several of these items are being sold under different labels.

Did I say that fresh and RTE foods are more likely to be contaminated? Four out of those six are RTE foods that we are likely to eat without cooking. (One of these items is sold by a nice, family-owned company that markets heavily to vegans and vegetarians.) Three could be carrying *L. monocytogenes,* which can be very serious for pregnant women and people with AIDS. The fourth RTE product is believed to be contaminated with *E. coli* O157:H7, which we all know can be deadly, particularly for young children. And this recall list shows only those contaminants for which testing is actually done, or which are present above permitted levels in our food. Many, many kinds of bacteria, parasites, low levels of mold toxins, chemicals, heavy metals, veterinary drug residues, or other toxic substances would never show up as a reason for a recall. So we blithely continue to ingest them, day after day, and year after year. The government only protects us to a certain extent. It can never keep our food supply completely safe. The rest is up to us.

It does not make sense to just sit back and wait for things to improve. I do not believe that this will happen over the next few years or decades. Unfortunately, there is no quick fix for our food system in spite of any government or industry efforts.

That leaves us with the Scout motto—"Be prepared." Or more specifically in this case, "Be informed and smart."

But you don't have to take my opinion. There are other scenarios for the future of our food. Let's try an optimistic one. Maybe instead, our food safety system will continually improve. Perhaps, after all, the budgets of food safety agencies will show major increase, and priorities, activities, and technology will be updated to twenty-first-century requirements. Our food-production environment may become cleaner as the worst POPs finally expire, cleanup efforts succeed, and industry becomes more environmentally conscious. Those nasty microbes such as *E. coli* O157:H7 and its toxin–producing relatives, those *Salmonella* species that seem to be everywhere, and those other bacteria, viruses, parasites, and molds we have talked about, may finally take fright and leave us alone. Or, maybe we'll find out that we—including our children—can thrive on any amount of nasty microbe toxins, toxic chemicals and metal residues in our food and live happily ever after, eating what we jolly well please.

I very much doubt it. I think another future scenario is much more likely. Let me describe it.

In future years, our domestically-grown food will become more and more mass produced, controlled by a limited number of producers and processors, as the smaller ones are progressively pushed out. Consolidation of small farms, processing facilities, food transporters, and distributors will continue. Such huge farming operations both home and abroad will need to use stronger pesticides, because insects, weeds, fungi, and other pests are increasing their resistance to those that are presently used. Larger amounts of synthetic fertilizer will be employed as soil becomes depleted by destructive farming practices. The irrigation water used for our fruits and vegetables will become further polluted. In spite of major efforts by those critical of such practices, there is a good chance that our meat and poultry will continue to be bombarded with drugs and hormones. More bacteria will become resistant to existing antibiotics, with subtherapeutic use of drugs for our meat animals and fish—and maybe even GM foods—playing a role in such growing resistance. The food we eat is likely to become more and more globalized, with an increasing proportion originating in countries that are not the safest for growing or processing food. Our farmed fish and shellfish—on which we are becoming increasingly reliant as ocean stocks become depleted—will become particularly unsafe to eat. So will our raw fruits and vegetables, and our increasingly popular and convenient ready-to-eat products.

Much as our government tries to identify and reject tainted food at our borders and to influence food quality and safety even before our trading partners send it to us, our imported food—even more than domestic food—will never be completely safe. Too many political and economic factors are involved.

Both large and small outbreaks in our food supply are likely to continue and be difficult to solve in spite of government efforts to promote better safety measures and trace-back procedures. Our food safety agencies will never have enough resources. Not nearly enough.

At the consumer end of the food system, the already existing eating trends will probably persist. Although there may be a temporary reversal during economic downturns that incline us to penny-pinch, over the longer term, we will increasingly dine outside the home. The lines between eating in and eating out will become blurred. We will buy more partially prepared or ready-to-eat produce, meats, poultry, fish, and baked goods for home meals, and eat more raw and minimally cooked foods when eating out. You could say this is the "worst of the worst" in terms of exposing us to food risks.

You don't need to just passively accept this situation, or go along with the usual trends. Nor do you need to live in daily fear of your food.

This is where the smart consumer enters the picture. You can become not just more nutrition conscious, but also more safety conscious. You could join those growing number of people who try to eat healthy food, organic food, local food, slow food, and sustainable food. (Safety aside, these foods also taste better.) You could join those who shop at farmers' markets, join community-supported agriculture ventures, have backyard or (now fashionable) front-yard gardens. Such eating styles will never fully protect you, but they will help to do so. Whatever you do, ultimately the safety of your food boils down to small, smart daily decisions and actions.

The informed consumer is an empowered consumer.

The empowered consumer can be a safe consumer.

You can be a safe consumer and still eat well.

Enjoy your food.

APPENDIX 1

Organizational Acronyms

ADA—American Dietetic Association

AMA—American Medical Association

ASTA—American Spice Trade Association

ATSDR—Agency for Toxic Substances and Disease Registry, a federal public health agency of New York Department of Health and Mental Hygiene (DOHMH)

CDC—United States Centers for Disease Control and Prevention (an agency of HHS)

CFIA—Canadian Food Inspection Agency

CFSAN—Center for Food Safety and Applied Nutrition (at FDA)

CRS—Congressional Research Service.

CVM—Center for Veterinary Medicine (at FDA)

DHHS—United States Department of Health and Human Services (often shortened to HHS)

EPA—Environmental Protection Agency

ERS—USDA's Economic Research Service

EU—European Union

FAO—United Nations Food and Agriculture Organization

FDA—United States Food and Drug Administration (an agency of HHS)

FSIS—Food Safety and Inspection Service (at USDA)

HC—Health Canada

HHS—United States Department of Health and Human Services

IARC—International Agency for Research on Cancer

JECFA—The Joint FAO/WHO Expert Committee on Food Additives

JEMRA—The Joint FA/WHO Expert Meeting on Microbiological Risk Assessment

JIFSAN—Joint Institute for Food Safety and Applied Nutrition

JIFSR—Joint Institute for Food Safety Research

IPCS—International Programme on Chemical Safety

NAS—National Academy of Sciences

NCEA—National Center for Environmental Assessment

USDA—United States Department of Agriculture

WHO—United Nations World Health Organization

| APPENDIX 2 |

Glossary

ADHD—Attention-deficit hyperactivity disorder is a neurobehavioral or developmental disorder that is characterized by a combination of attention problems and hyperactivity. There are several subtypes. ADHD is more common among boys. Often diagnosed in children, it can persist through adulthood. Exact cause is still unknown.

AFLATOXIN—A common mycotoxin typically produced by the fungus *Aspergillus flavus,* which can be present on such crops as peanuts, tree nuts, and corn, and even fruits and vegetables. The levels of aflatoxin in our food are regulated by the FDA. If animals such as milk cattle are given aflatoxin-contaminated feed, this toxin can also be present in their milk.

ANIMAL PRODUCTS—Animal products are either produced by an animal or taken from the body of an animal. They include dairy, seafood, eggs, honey, and meat, as well as many more animal-derived ingredients such as gelatin and casein. See vegetarian and vegan Web sites for a more complete list.

ANTIBIOTICS—Powerful medicines that kill bacteria or keep them from reproducing. Antibiotics do not work against viruses. Most antibiotics are made of natural substances such as bacteria or molds (fungi). The term was originally used to only describe substances made from such living organisms, but is now often also applied to a few synthetic substances—that is, made completely in the laboratory—such as sulfonamides.

ANTIBIOTIC RESISTANCE—The ability of a microorganism to withstand the effects of an antibiotic or several antibiotics that are designed to work on it. If a strain of bacteria is resistant to a wide range of antibiotics, then it is sometimes referred to as a "superbug." Overuse and misuse of antibiotics, as in livestock production, can contribute to development of antibiotic resistance to similar drugs in humans, but antibiotic resistance in human pathogens is also due to the overuse or misuse of antibiotics in human medicine.

ANTIBIOTIC SENSITIVITY—A bacteria is sensitive to an antibiotic if that antibiotic kills it or limits its growth. Sensitivity analysis in the laboratory can be done to see which antibiotic is likely to be most effective. Some antibiotics work better on one type of bacteria than on others. Bacteria can lose their sensitivity to antibiotics over time.

ANTIMICROBIAL—A broad, umbrella term, referring to all kinds of natural, semisynthetic, or synthetic substances, including medicines, lotions, sprays or other products that are used to slow down or kill microorganisms (bacteria, viruses, parasites, and fungi). Antimicrobials include antibiotics, antivirals, antiparasitic drugs, and antifungals.

AVIAN INFLUENZA—A viral infection, commonly known as "bird flu," caused by H5N1 virus. Outbreaks in birds were first reported in 1996 in China, but the virus has since spread around the world and affected animals and humans as well as wild and domestic birds. The virus has proven resistant to common antiviral drugs. The fatality rate is very high.

BACTERIA–Sometimes referred to as "bugs," are simple and extremely small organisms—usually 0.3 to 2.0 micrometers in diameter—which multiply very rapidly and can survive under a wide range of conditions. Bacteria exist in large numbers in soil, water, and the skin and digestive tracts of humans and animals. Upper-end estimates of the total number of species of bacteria range from ten million to a billion, but no one really knows. The "good" bacteria include those useful in helping digest our food and protecting us from disease. Other bacteria are "pathogenic"; that is, they can cause disease in humans and/or animals.

BIOACCUMULATION–Refers to a process whereby concentrations of a chemical increase in the body over time, with more stored than is metabolized or excreted. For additional explanation of the process, see: http://extoxnet.orst.edu/tibs/bioaccum.htm.

BODY BURDEN–The chemical load of harmful substances that have accumulated in a person's body. This quantity, measured usually in the blood or urine, is expressed in units such as grams or milligrams.

BOTULISM–A particularly deadly form of food poisoning, less common these days, caused by the ingestion of a food or drink contaminated with the toxin produced by the bacterium *Clostridium botulinum*.

BSE–Bovine spongiform encephalopathy, the technical name for "mad cow disease." It is a form of transmissible spongiform encephalopathy (TSE), a group of progressive, incurable, and very dangerous diseases caused by prions (see *prions*) These diseases can be transmitted between mammals when one mammal eats a part of the nervous system of another which is diseased. BSE is found in cattle, scrapie is the TSE associated with sheep, and feline spongiform encephalopathy (FSE) is the version in cats. Kuru, a human version, once occurred among the South Foré of Papua New Ginea, spread by eating dead relatives during ritual funerary practices.

CANCER HEALTH RISK—The Environmental Protection Agency (EPA) classifies substances as Class A, Class B, Class C, Class D, or Class E, in terms of their ability to cause cancer in humans and animals. Class A substances are "known" human carcinogens, Class B "probable" human carcinogens, and Class C "possible" human carcinogens.

CARCINOGEN—A substance or organism that is known to cause cancer in humans or animals, increase the chances of the occurrence of cancer, or aggravate existing cancer. Some may occur naturally in food, for instance, when it is cooked; others are introduced into foods via contact with toxic chemicals or metals during farming, storage, or food processing. Certain microbial toxins, hormones, and viruses have also been found to promote cancer in humans as well as in animals. Carcinogens normally cause cancer only after a long period of exposure—as long as several decades, but sometimes much less. The type of carcinogen involved, its levels, and the duration of exposure are likely to influence cancer occurrence.

CARDIOVASCULAR—Pertaining to the heart and blood vessels.

CHLORDANE—A toxic chemical that was used as a pesticide in the United States from 1948 to 1988 on crops such as corn and citrus, until banned by the FDA. Chlordane can persist in the soil for over twenty years. It can build up in the tissues of fish, birds, and mammals.

COMMUNITY SUPPORTED AGRICULTURE (CSA)—A farm that is supported by a group or "community" of people who share the financial risks by paying a membership fee and are then entitled to a share of the fresh-picked produce (and sometimes other agricultural products) during the growing season. When it works well, this arrangement benefits both the farmer and the participating consumers.

CONVENTIONAL AGRICULTURE—A system of agriculture that is characterized by reliance on a very small number of crops, on mechanization, and use of synthetic inputs such as chemical fertilizers and pesticides. This system stresses productivity and profitability with little attention to sustainability. Modern industrialized agriculture is mainly conventional agriculture, although more and more industrialized producers are now also engaging in organic production.

COOKING CHEMICALS—Chemicals formed in food under high-heat conditions during cooking. Toxic cooking chemicals are sometimes also referred to as "cooking contaminants." Some cooking chemicals are known, probable, or possible carcinogens.

CONTAMINANT—A substance that is present where it does not belong, or is present at higher levels than allowed, which might cause harm.

CREUTZFELDT-JAKOB DISEASE (CJD)—A rare human encephalopathy, the new variant of which is believed to be contracted through eating BSE-contaminated beef.

CROSS-CONTAMINATION—The transfer of contaminants from one food source (such as raw meat, poultry, or eggs) to another (such as salads or cooked food). This can occur in a number of ways, usually through contaminated cutting tools, dishes, unwashed hands, or even directly if foods are placed next to each other.

DDT—Dichloro diphenyl trichloroethane, a highly toxic insecticide, which bioaccumulates in the body. It is now banned in the United States but still present in the environment.

DIELDRIN—A persistent chlorinated hydrocarbon, a by-product of the insecticide Aldrin. It is highly toxic and bioaccumulates in the body. It was previously widely used to control insects on corn and citrus crops. Most uses are now banned in America. Dieldrin has been linked to Parkinson's syndrome.

DEMOIC ACID—A deadly neurotoxin associated with amnesic shellfish poisoning. It originates in red algae and can be very deadly to the elderly.

DIARRHEA—Frequent discharge of watery stools. Diarrhea may be caused by microbial, parasitic, or viral infections, or other factors.

DOSE—The amount of a substance that a person is exposed to. When referring to amounts of a toxic substance in food, the "dose" is usually stated in terms of milligram per kilogram of body weight per day.

EMULSIFIER—A substance added to products, such as meat spreads, to prevent separation of product components and ensure consistency. Examples of such additives include lecithin and mono- and diglycerides.

ENVIRONMENTAL CONTAMINANTS—Toxic substances that get into food as a result of hazardous waste or industrial pollution of the soil, water, or air. For recent studies of specific ones and more general information, consult www.cdc.gov/exposurereport/.

FOOD ADDITIVES—Substances added to food. *Direct* food additives are added to food for a specific purpose, such as preventing spoilage, improving or maintaining nutritional value, or making the food product more attractive by enhancing taste, texture, or color. The most common food additives (if measured by quantity) are flavorings, which include spices, vinegar, synthetic flavors, and particularly sweeteners. *Indirect* food additives end up in the food in very small amounts as a result of packaging, storage or handling. (For more information: www.foodsafety.gov/~lrd/foodaddi. html.)

FOOD-BORNE ILLNESS, OR FOOD POISONING—A gastrointestinal illness, usually caused by eating, but sometimes also by handling contaminated food. There are over 250 possible causes, maybe even thousands. Although the terms are used in various ways, in its widest sense they includes two main types of contaminants: microorganisms (bacteria, viruses, parasites, and fungi) and toxic agents (such as natural toxins and environmental chemicals). Food-borne illness varies considerably in its severity, and to some extent also in its onset, duration, and symptoms. Common symptoms are nausea, vomiting, abdominal cramps, and diarrhea. Skin lesions, headache, and fever can occur with certain types. The most usual onset is twelve to thirty-six hours after eating, but it can be as little as thirty minutes. (See the Mayo Clinic Web site for common kinds of food-borne illness and their symptoms.)

FOOD CONTACT SUBSTANCES—Substances that have contact with food. They include coatings, plastics, paper, adhesives, colorants, antimicrobials, and antioxidants. The responsibilities of the U.S. Food and Drug Administration's (FDA) Center for Food Safety and Applied Nutrition (CFSAN) include regulating industry to make sure that food contact substances are safe. Because this is such a huge and separate topic, most relevant in the case of processed foods, which are not the focus of this book, it is not discussed.

FOOD HAZARD—A potentially harmful natural or artificial substance in food that is reasonably likely to cause human illness or injury. There is a wide range of potential food hazards, including microorganisms, naturally present chemicals, chemicals produced by cooking, environmental contaminants, additives, and pesticides.

FOOD-SERVICE INDUSTRY—The restaurant and food catering business.

FOOD TERRORISM—Refers to the sabotage of food sabotage by terrorists or other criminals. Some of the "weapons" that could be used include bacteria like *Bacillus anthracis* (anthrax) and *Clostridium botulinum* (botulism), *Salmonella* spp., *Shigella dysenteriae, E. coli* O157:H7, and ricin. Some of these are also involved in the unintentional contamination of food. Natural plant toxins, such as ricin, and industrial chemicals, such as melamine, are other possible weapons of food sabotage. (More information: http://www.cfsan.fda.gov/~dms/rabtact.html#ii)

FRESH-CUT PRODUCE—Fresh fruit or vegetables that have been minimally processed prior to packaging and sale, usually including washing and one or more of the following: peeling, slicing, chopping, shredding, coring, or trimming (e.g., precut, packaged, ready-to-eat salads). Fresh-cut produce does not usually need additional preparation, processing, or cooking before it is eaten.

FRESH PRODUCE—Fruit or vegetables that are sold in an unprocessed (i.e., raw) form.

FUMONISIN—A kind of mycotoxin produced by fungi ("molds") in the genus *Fusarium. Fusarium moniliforme* (*Fusarium verticillioides*) is commonly found in corn.

FUNGI—Commonly referred to as "molds"—but the group actually includes molds, yeasts, and mushrooms. Fungi are living organisms, with nuclei, which are distantly related to plants. Fungi usually reproduce by means of spores. Some fungi are edible, but others produce toxins that are very deadly to humans.

GASTROINTESTINAL (GI)—Involving the stomach and small and large intestines.

GASTROENTERITIS—Inflammation of the intestine and stomach. It is a common disorder, and can range from mild to severe, and even fatal (in the elderly). Usual symptoms are vomiting, diarrhea, and abdominal discomfort.

GENETICALLY MODIFIED ORGANISMS—An organism that has been genetically altered by the transfer of DNA from another organism.

GRASS-FED—The reliance on pasture or rangeland to feed livestock. In this situation, grazing and forage feeding replaces high-grain diets, close confinement, and feedlot finishing during most or all of the animals' lifetime.

HACCP—Abbreviation for Hazard Analysis and Critical Control Point procedures. HACCP is a food safety approach, used in several countries, including the United States and Canada, which calls for food industries to implement preventive measures based on identification of key points in the systems where hazards are most likely to enter.

IMMUNE SYSTEM—A network of cells, organs, and tissues that work together to protect the body against the attacks of foreign "invaders."

INDUSTRIAL CHEMICALS—Chemicals manufactured for use in industrial operations or research.

INFECTIVE DOSE—The number of organisms that make individuals ill or carriers. Several different factors will affect this number.

INGESTION—The act of swallowing something via eating or drinking it.

INORGANIC—Compounds composed of mineral materials, including elemental salts and metals such as iron, aluminum, mercury, and zinc.

INTEGRATED PEST MANAGEMENT (IPM)—An ecologically based approach to pest control in agriculture, which relies on close understanding of the pests themselves and of pest-crop relationships and minimizes risk to human health and the environment. It tends to use a combination of techniques such as habitat manipulation, use of resistant varieties, and biological control. IPM is a labor-intensive approach to controlling crop pests, which can reduce or even eliminate the need for pesticides.

IRRADIATION—The process of exposing food to ionizing radiation for the purpose of destroying microorganisms. Food irradiation is currently allowed to a greater or lesser extent by over 40 countries, including the United States.

LOCALLY PRODUCED—Depending on who is using the concept, the definition of "local" can vary from a relatively small area to the size of an entire state. One popular definition is "no farther than a normal day's drive" for a transport truck (about 400 miles). Unfortunately, often goods that are marketed as "locally produced" have actually been grown or processed at a distance of thousands of miles, and simply packaged or repackaged locally. Some large retailers define any food they sell as "local" if it is grown in the same state as it is sold.

LOCAVORE—Also known as "localvore"; a word coined in 2005 by four women (some reports credit one woman) in San Francisco, meaning someone who prefers to eat locally harvested food. Often, this is defined as within a 100-mile radius, but sometimes greater. The locavore movement encourages consumers to buy from farmers' markets or even to grow or pick their own food, maintaining that fresh, local products are more nutritious and taste better. Related term: "local food movement."

LOW-INPUT PRACTICES—The minimal use by farmers of external inputs such as purchased fertilizer and pesticides, with reliance on on-farm use of organic materials and IPM practices (see *Integrated pest management*). In theory, this approach would lower costs to the farmer, lower environmental pollution, and lower levels of chemicals in food, but it can also lower productivity.

MAD COW DISEASE—See *BSE*.

MELAMINE—A toxic industrial chemical used to make a wide variety of products such as plastics, glues, coatings, paint, certain insecticides, and food packaging.

MERCURY—A heavy metal that occurs in the environment in different chemical forms, most commonly metallic mercury, mercuric sulfide, mercuric chloride and methyl mercury. Mercury can be found in nearly all fish, to a greater or lesser degree. It has also been found in very small amounts in a number of other foods—including ones often preferred by children—such as some corn syrup, chocolate syrup, cereal bars, yogurt, jelly, and soft drinks.

MICROBE, OR MICROORGANISM—A collective name given to bacteria, parasites, fungi, and viruses. Microbes are living organisms that are masters at adapting to their environment and surviving. They are everywhere—in our environment, on our skin, and in our body. Some serve useful functions, others can be harmful, and many can become harmful under certain circumstances, such as when sufficient numbers of pathogenic microbes are transferred from the soil to our mouth.

MOLDS—See *fungi*.

MYCOTOXIN—Metabolic by-products of fungi that are toxic to animals and humans. Not all fungi produce them, and the ones that do only do so under certain conditions. The best-known mycotoxin is aflatoxin.

NATURAL TOXINS—Potentially harmful substances that are produced by a particular plant or animal. Some are always present, whereas others only develop if the plant or animal is damaged or threatened. Examples are mushroom toxins and toxins in fish.

ORGANIC FARMING—The USDA Study Team on Organic Farming defines it as: "a production system which avoids or largely excludes the use of synthetically compounded fertilizers, pesticides, growth regulators, and livestock feed additives. To the maximum extent feasible, organic farming systems rely upon crop rotations, crop residues, animal manures, legumes, green manures, off-farm organic wastes, mechanical cultivation, mineral-bearing rocks, and aspects of biological pest control to maintain soil productivity and tilth, to supply plant nutrients, and to control insects, weeds and other pests." (More information: www.misa.umn.edu/vd/bull.ppt.)

ORGANIC FOOD—Food that is produced without using most conventional pesticides, fertilizers made with synthetic ingredients or sewage sludge, bioengineering, or irradiation. To be truly organic, poultry, meat, dairy, or egg products have to come from animals that are not given growth hormones or regular subtherapeutic doses of antibiotics. The U.S. government requires that any products labeled "organic" meet a set of strict conditions and obtain certification. Companies that handle organic food also need to meet defined organic standards. See http://www.ams.usda.gov/AMSv1.0/nop.

OUTBREAK—When applied to food-borne illness, this term means that two or more people who have eaten the same contaminated food have become ill. Larger and/or more widespread outbreaks are due to contamination of food early on in the food chain (for instance, during production, harvesting or processing). Smaller ones tend to result from contamination of food in a restaurant, school, jail, or similar group setting; at a social event; or in the home. The numbers of illnesses reported in larger outbreaks can be assumed to represent only a very small fraction of the actual cases of illness that have occurred.

PARASITES—Organisms that live on or inside another organism, on which they feed. There are thousands of parasites of different kinds and sizes, some looking almost like earthworms and others being single-cell protozoa. Human parasites can be carried by food and water. They cause not only short-term illness but also multiple longer-term health problems, because they not only steal nutrients from the body but also secrete toxins. (For more information: http://www.fsis.usda.gov/factsheets/parasites _and_foodborne_illness/index.asp, or http://www.appliedozone .com/parasites.html.)

PATHOGENIC–Capable of causing illness or death.

PATHOGENS–Organisms that cause illness or death, such as bacteria, viruses, and parasites. A common way that pathogens enter the body is through the mouth, as when contaminated food is eaten. There is a period of time (ranging from hours to days) between the time the pathogen enters and the time the person begins to feel ill. There are also cases where healthy people have ingested pathogens but have had mild or no symptoms at all.

PCBS–Polychlorinated biphenyls, which are a type of man-made organic chemical that in the past was used in hundreds of commercial and industrial products. PCBs can cause cancer as well as have several other types of adverse health effects. Their manufacture was banned in the United States in 1979 because of their toxic nature, but once in the environment, PCBs do not break down readily and can therefore still contaminate our food.

PESTICIDES–Chemical or biological products that have been developed with the purpose of controlling weeds, insects, fungi, diseases, or other pests on crops, on animals, or in the environment (places such as schools, hospitals, nursing homes, and parks). The most common pesticides are insecticides (used to control insects), fungicides (used to control molds or fungi), herbicides (used to control weeds), molluscicides (used to control slugs and snails), and rodenticides (used to control rats and mice). In food production, most—but not all—pesticides are used during the production stage.

POP—"Persistent organic pollutants" are man-made toxic chemicals either once approved for use in agriculture, industry, manufacture, or control of disease (such as malaria), or produced unintentionally by industrial processes or by combustion. They can bioaccumulate in the body and persist in the environment for long periods of time (sometimes decades). Both the United States and Canada have taken strong action to control POPs.

PRION—Tiny protein particles believed to be the cause of BSE.

PROCESSING WATER—Water used for postharvest handling of produce, such as washing, cooling, waxing, or product transport.

PROTOZOA—A very small single-celled organisms, with a nucleus, surrounded by a nuclear membrane. It can be seen only under a microscope. Protozoa can be found almost anywhere on earth. About 20 percent of the known fifty thousand protozoa are parasitic; that is, they can feed upon vertebrates and invertebrates; some even infect plants. Some parasitic protozoa have very complex life cycles and several "hosts."

RECALL—The removal of designated food (or other) products from the marketplace or from other client companies to which they may have been sent. Main reasons for food recalls are adulteration (contamination) or misbranding (under the provisions of existing laws). The government classifies recalls according to their level of health risk, from Class I (most severe) to Class III.

RISK—The probability of an adverse event occurring.

SEROVAR—Means the same as "strain" of bacteria, and is short for "serological variant."

SHIGA TOXIN (OR SHIGA-LIKE TOXIN) – A deadly toxin produced by certain bacteria, such as *Shigella disenteriae* and Shiga-like toxin–producing *Escherichia coli* (STEC). Among the many STEC serotypes, *E. coli* O157:H7 is the most frequently reported.

SUPERBUGS – Bacteria that are resistant to almost all antibiotics. Such bacteria are increasing in number and are a major global public health threat.

SUSTAINABLY PRODUCED – When applied to food production, this concept usually implies that the food has been grown with responsible use of natural resources (such as soil, water, and biodiversity), with reduced energy consumption and with care to reduce negative impact, such as by greenhouse gases or overuse of chemicals. However, frequently the concept also carries a range of animal and human welfare, economic, social, and health implications.

SUSTAINABLE AGRICULTURE – This concept is normally used to refer to an agriculture system that could be maintained indefinitely. In its broad use, the term implies that the agriculture system will be not only ecologically sound but also economically viable over the longer term, and socially just.

SYNTHETIC – Produced artificially or "man-made."

SYNTHETIC FERTILIZER – Fertilizer made with artificially made ingredients, such as urea, ammonia, and ammonium sulfate. These are usually by-products of the oil and natural gas industry.

SUBTHERAPEUTIC – Below the dosage levels used to treat diseases. In livestock production, antibiotics are frequently used at subtherapeutic levels to improve animal growth rates and feed efficiency.

TOXIC – A substance that has the power to be harmful, poisonous, or destructive when swallowed, inhaled, or absorbed through the skin is toxic. Some toxins are naturally occurring, whereas others are man-made. (For more information and answers to common questions consult http://www.atsdr.cdc.gov/tfacts35.html.)

TRIANGULATION—A social science research technique that helps to overcome biases, weaknesses, or research errors that may occur if relying on a single source for conclusions. In essence, it validates data through cross-verification from more than two sources, often selecting those studies using different approaches or methodologies, or that started with a different hypothesis or viewpoint. It can be used in quantitative or qualitative studies. Triangulation was used in writing this book.

VIRUS—A submicroscopic infectious agent, smaller than bacteria, which can only grow and reproduce in a host. About five thousand viruses have been described, but many more remain undiscovered. Viruses can also exist in food products and cause disease in humans, but some of them, known as "bacteriophages" (viruses that infect bacteria), are also being used to protect foods against dangerous bacteria (as when a virus cocktail is sprayed on meat or poultry to protect it from *Listeria* backteria).

VOMITOXIN—Also called "deoxynivalenol (DON)," a mycotoxin produced primarily by the fungi *Fusarium graminearum* and *F. culmorum*. It occurs mainly in grains such as barley, oats, maize and wheat, and occasionally in rice and sorghum. A number of factors are involved in whether the fungus produces this toxin. Compared to many other mycotoxins, vomitoxin is relatively mild in its effects on livestock or humans.

Getting Help

To Check Food Safety Alerts

United States

- To check current USAID recalls (meat, poultry, and egg products): http://www.fsis.usda.gov/FSIS_Recalls/Open _Federal_Cases/index.asp.
- To check current FDA recalls (all except meat, poultry, or egg products): http://www.fda.gov/safety/recalls/ default.htm.
- To check on a toxic substance, contact the Agency for Toxic Substances and Disease Registry (ATSDR): http://www.atsdr.cdc.gov/.
- Fish advisories: http://www.epa.gov/waterscience/fish/ states.htm.

Canada

- To check current CFIA high-alert recalls: http://www .inspection.gc.ca/english/corpaffr/recarapp/recaltoce.shtml.

To Report a Problem with Food or Obtain Emergency Help

United States

- CDC's 24/7 hotline: 1-800-232-4346/TTY / 1-888-232-6348, or cdcinfo@cdc.gov.
- Concerning meat, poultry, or liquid eggs, USAID/FSIS's hotline: 1-888-674-6854 or 1-800-535-4555.
- For emergencies concerning any food *except* meat; poultry; or frozen, dried, or liquid eggs: FDA's emergency hotline at 301-443-1240. For complaints that are not urgent, check the FDA's Web site to find the contact telephone number of your local consumer complaint coordinator: http://www.fda.gov/Safety/ReportaProblem/Consumer ComplaintCoordinators/default.htm.
- For a toxic substance emergency, including in food, call ATSDR's Emergency Response Hotline (24 hours): 404-498-0120. For general information on a toxic sub-stance: 1-888-422-8737.
- Concerning pesticides, contact the National Pesticide Information Center (7 days a week, 6:30 AM–4:30 AM PT): 1-800-858-7378 or e-mail npic@ace.orst.edu.
- For issues with products sold online: webcomplaints@ ora.fda.gov.

Canada

- CFIA's emergency response hotline: 1-800-442-2342 / 1-613-225-2342 / TTY 1-800-465-7735.
- To ask a nonemergency question online: http://www .inspection.gc.ca/english/tools/feedback/commene.shtml.
- Concerning chemical contaminants in food: www.hc-sc .gc.ca/contact/fn-an/hpfb-dgpsa/bmhr-bdmr-eng.php.

- For information on microbial food-related illnesses (Bureau of Microbial Hazards): http://www.hc-sc.gc.ca/contact/fn-an/hpfb-dgpsa/bmhr-bdmr-eng.php.

To Contact Government Agencies or Search Their Web Sites

United States

Agency for Toxic Substances and Disease Registry (ATSDR)
4770 Buford Hwy, NE
Atlanta, GA 30341
Phone: 1-800-232-4636
TTY: 1-888-232-6348
http://www.atsdr.cdc.gov
To locate your regional office:
    http://www.atsdr.cdc.gov/DRO/index.html

Center for Food Safety and Applied Nutrition (FDA/CFSAN)
5100 Paint Branch Parkway
College Park, MD 20740–3835
Food information line: 1-888-SAFEFOOD (1-888-723-3366)
http://www.cfsan.fda.gov

Centers for Disease Control and Prevention (CDC)
1600 Clifton Road
Atlanta, GA 30333
General information: 1-800-232-4636
http://www.cdc.gov

USDA Food Safety and Inspection Service (USDA/FSIS)
U.S. Department of Agriculture
Washington, D.C. 20250-3700
Phone: 1-888-674-6854
http://www.fsis.usda.gov

U.S. Department of Health and Human Services (HHS)
200 Independence Avenue SW
Washington, D.C. 20201
Phone: 1-877-696-6775 or 202-619-0257
http://www.os.dhhs.gov

U.S. Environmental Protection Agency (EPA)
Ariel Rios Building
1200 Pennsylvania Avenue NW
Washington, D.C. 20460
Phone: 202–272–0167
http://www.epa.gov

U.S. Food and Drug Administration (FDA)
FDA (HFE-88)
5600 Fishers Lane
Rockville, MD 20857-0001
General inquiries: 1-888-463-6332
http://www. fda.gov

Canada

Bureau of Chemical Safety
Health Products and Food Branch
Health Canada
Sir Frederick Banting Research Centre
Postal Locator: 2203B
Ottawa, Ontario K1A 0L2
Phone: 1-800-267-1245/613-957-0973
http://www.hc-sc.gc.ca

Bureau of Microbial Hazards
Sir F. G. Banting Research Centre
Postal Locator 2204A2
Tunney's Pasture
Ottawa, Ontario
K1A 0L2
Phone: 1-800-267-1245 / 613-957-0908
http://www.hc-sc.gc.ca

Canadian Food Inspection Agency (CFIA)
(National Headquarters)
Canadian Food Inspection Agency
1400 Merivale Road
Ottawa, Ontario
K1A 0Y9
Phone: 1-800-442-2342 / 613-225-2342
http://www.cfia.gov

CFIA Area Offices

To locate your area office address and telephone numbers: http://www
.inspection.gc.ca/english/directory/offbure.shtml

Health Canada (HC)

Health Canada
Brooke Claxton Building, Tunney's Pasture
Postal Locator: 0906C
Ottawa, Ontario K1A 0K9
Phone: 1-866-225-0709 / 613-957-2991
http://www.hc-sc.gc.ca

| **APPENDIX 4** |

Further Reading

THOUSANDS OF SOURCES were used for this book during more than three years of research. This section can only list a small sample. It gives priority to those that are easy to read and access online.

General Background Reading

Online Information

- Tailored advice, if you are in a high-risk group (have cancer, diabetes, are older, or other): http://www.fsis. usda.gov/factsheets/At_Risk_&_Underserved_Fact _Sheets/index.asp.
- General background about bacteria in relation to food: http://www.fsis.usda.gov/PDF/PHVt-Food_Microbiology .pdf, or http://digestive.niddk.nih.gov/ddiseases/pubs/ bacteria/.

    An overview of progress in dealing with common bacteria in our food supply: http://www.cdc.gov/mmwr/ preview/mmwrhtml/mm5813a2.htm.
- About antibiotic resistance: http://www.cdc.gov/ drugresistance/.

For details on progress and results of ongoing government research: http://www.cdc.gov/drugresistance/actionplan/2008report/Inventory_of_Projects_AR2008_01152010_final.pdf.

■ An overview of parasites in food-borne illness: http://www.fsis.usda.gov/Fact_Sheets/Parasites_and_Foodborne_Illness/index.aspan.

For those who are brave: http://members.cox.net/llyee/detecting_microbes.html.

■ An overview of the protozoan parasites: http://www.safewater.org/PDFS/resourcesknowthefacts/Protozoan_Parasites.pdf.

■ An overview of viruses, especially norovirus: http://www.cdc.gov/ncidod/dvrd/revb/gastro/norovirus-foodhandlers.htm.

A practical summary of viral gastroenteritis (often called "stomach flu"): http://www.clemson.edu/extension/hgic/food/food_safety/illnesses/hgic3720.html.

■ An overview of molds in food: http://www.fsis.usda.gov/factsheets/molds_on_food/, or http://ucce.ucdavis.edu/files/repositoryfiles/ca3311p18-62692.pdf.

■ An overview of pesticides and history of their use in the United States: http://ipm.ncsu.edu/safety/factsheets/pestuse.pdf.

Pesticides residues in U.S. food (updated): http://cfpub.epa.gov/eroe/index.cfm?fuseaction=detail.viewPDF&ch=48&lShowInd=0&subtop=312&lv=list.listByChapter&r=188237. To check on tolerances for those "unavoidable" poisons in your favorite foods: http://www.fda.gov/Food/GuidanceComplianceRegulatoryInformation/GuidanceDocuments/ChemicalContaminantsand Pesticides/ucm077969.htm.

■ An overview of heavy metals: http://www.lenntech.com/processes/heavy/heavy-metals/heavy-metals.htm.

■ A list of the twelve POPs: http://www.ewg.org/node/19443.

- An objective look at irradiation: http://www.fsis.usda.gov/ Fact_Sheets/Irradiation_and_Food_Safety/index.asp.

General Books on Food Safety You May Want to Read

Entis, Phyllis. *Food Safety: Old Habits and New Perspectives.* American Society of Microbiology, 2008. A more technical book, focusing on water as well as food, with light touches and many useful sections.

Fox, Nicols. *It Was Probably Something You Ate.* Penguin Books, 1999. Written by an intelligent journalist who became fascinated by microorganisms in food, particularly bacteria.

Mindell, Earl, and Hester Mundis. *Unsafe at Any Meal.* Contemporary Books, written in 1987, updated in 2002. Good for looking up specific processed foods for a quick scare-bite, especially from a nutritional perspective. The book covers a huge range of topics, including additives and packaging, with no shades of gray.

Nestle, Marion. *What To Eat.* North Point Press, 2007. A very informative and readable book by a leading nutritionist. Covers topics broader than food safety and includes useful shopping information.

Satin, Morton. *Food Alert.* Checkmark Books, 1999. Good information for self-diagnosis and some delightfully grue-some (but useful) illustrations.

Winter, Ruth. *Poisons in Your Food*, rev. ed. Crown Publishers, Inc., 1990. Written by the pioneer of food safety in the United States and still worth reading.

Suggested Reading to Supplement Topics Covered by This Book

On Genetically Modified Food

- For a good, but ultimately positive, overview of the issue, available online: http://www.biosci.utexas.edu/ib/faculty/jansen/FS301%20papers/Oeschger_Silva.pdf.
- A readable and useful book, although the field has changed a bit since its publication: Ronnie Cummins and Ben Lilliston, *Genetically Engineered Food: A Self-Defense Guide for Consumers* (Marlowe and Co., 2000).
- A must-read on GM—if you have the courage: Jeffrey M. Smith, *Seeds of Deception: Exposing Government Deception and Lies About the Safety of the Genetically Modified Foods You're Eating* (Chelsea Green Publishing, 2007).
- For a more recent view of the issue: Lisa H. Weasel, *Food Fray: Inside the Controversy on Genetically Modified Food* (AMACOM, 2009).

On Safety Issues in Processed Foods

- An online source of various reports and articles: http://www.cspinet.org/reports/.
- For the FDA's reassuring view of additives: http://www.fda.gov/food/foodingredientspackaging/ucm094211.htm.
- For a quick read on the risks: Paula Johanson, *What's In Your Food? Recipe for Disaster* (Rosen Central, 2008).
- An excellent guide for consumers who read labels, this book gives the facts about relative safety and any side effects of some eight thousand additives that turn up in our food as a result of processing. Ruth Winter, *A Consumer's Dictionary of Food Additives* (Three Rivers Press, 1999 [updated edition]).

On Supplements

- For a comprehensive view of products available in the United States and Canada: Lyle MacWilliam, *A Comparative Guide to Nutritional Supplements* (Northern Dimensions Publishing, 2003).
- A comprehensive overview, but with some advice that you should double-check for differing opinions: Phyllis Balch and James Balch, *Prescription to Nutritional Healing* (Balch Books, 2008).
- For a readable lowdown on herbal and nutritional supplements as well as other issues: Dr. Arthur Winter and Ruth Winter, *Smart Food: Diet and Nutrition for Maximum Brain Power* (Universe Inc., 2007 [originally published in 1999]).
- If you have diabetes: Laura Shane-McWhorter, *Guide to Herbs and Nutritional Supplements for Diabetes* (The American Diabetes Association, 2009).

Fruits and Vegetables

Microbes

- A comprehensive overview of the issue: Jennylynd James, *Microbial Hazard Identification in Fresh Fruits and Vegetables* (John Wiley and Sons, Inc., 2006).
- Why unpasteurized juices and ciders are risky: http://www.healthlinkbc.ca/healthfiles/hfile72.stm.

Pesticides

- For reliable summary information on any pesticide, search EXTOXNET: (http://extoxnet.orst.edu). EXTOXNET is a collaborative effort between several leading U.S. universities with a strong agriculture focus.
- Particularly for those concerned about children's exposure to pesticide residues: "Pesticides and Children: NAS Report Sets Table to Serve Up Policy Changes" (National Academy

of Sciences report on pesticides in children's diets): http://www.nap.edu/openbook.php?isbn=0309048753.

- For the research on the link between organophosphates and ADHD: http://pediatrics.aappublications.org/cgi/content/abstract/peds.2009-3058v1.
- A reasoned argument in favor of safer organic foods, especially for children: http://www.biotech-info.net/Ecofarm_Food_Safety.pdf.

Molds

- A technical discussion of the mycotoxin issue: Barry G. Swanson, *Mycotoxins on Fruits and Vegetables,* available on the Web site of the International Society for Horticultural Science (ISHS), http://www.actahort.org/books/207/207_5.htm.

Parasites

- A good overview of human parasites, including ones linked to produce: http://www.aafp.org/afp/2004/0301/p1161.html.
- A summary of the *Cyclospora*/raspberry case: http://www.innovations-report.de/html/berichte/agrar_forstwissenschaften/bericht-109179.html or the IFPRI account on http://www.ifpri.org/2020/focus/focus10/focus10_07.pdf.
- Additional information on the *Toxoplasma* parasite: http://www.cdc.gov/toxoplasmosis/factsheet.html#what.

Mushroom Toxins

- A comprehensive FDA online source of information on mushroom toxins: http://www.foodsafety.gov/~mow/chap40.html.
- For more technical information, plus pictures: the *National Audubon Society Field Guide to Mushrooms—North America* (Alfred A. Knopf, 2001), which covers more than seven

hundred species. (It also has a great cooking section.) This book is a must for anyone who collects wild mushrooms.

■ The basics on oxalates: http://www.whfoods.com/genpage .php?tname=george&dbid=48.

Acrylamide

■ The FDA position on the issue: http://www.fda.gov/ Food/FoodSafety/FoodContaminantsAdulteration/ ChemicalContaminants/Acrylamide/ucm053519.htm.

■ A cautiously worded industry overview of the issue: http://www.acrylamidefacts.org/.

Irradiation

■ A quick, although dated, overview on the basics of produce irradiation: http://www.aphis.usda.gov/publications/ plant_health/content/printable_version/ifruit08.pdf.

■ An entirely negative view of irradiation: http://www .foodandwaterwatch.org/.

Fish and Shellfish

Bacteria and Viruses

■ A good comprehensive review, but with very outdated illness patterns and statistics: http://seafood.ucdavis.edu/ Pubs/safety1.htm.

■ A practical summary of main causes of illness and risk factors: http://www.clemson.edu/extension/hgic/food/ food_safety/illnesses/hgic3660.html.

■ A must-read for anyone who loves oysters: http://www .issc.org/client_resources/Education/VvFactSheet.pdf.

Parasites

■ A quick practical review of parasites in marine fish: http://seagrant.oregonstate.edu/sgpubs/onlinepubs/ g03015.pdf.

- An introduction to freshwater fish parasites: http://edis
  .ifas.ufl.edu/fa041.

Natural Toxins

- Practical information on scromboid poisoning: http://
  www.clemson.edu/extension/hgic/food/food_safety/
  illnesses/hgic3662.html.
- Practical information on ciguatera poisoning: http://
  www.clemson.edu/extension/hgic/food/pdf/hgic3661.
  pdf.

Dangerous Drugs

- Drugs used in U.S. aquaculture: http://aquanic.org/
  species/catfish/documents/Drugs_and_Chemicals_in
  _US_Aquaculture_11.10.pdf.
- A government report, which includes findings on
  fluoroquinolone-resistant bacteria from imported
  shrimp: http://www.cdc.gov/drugresistance/actionplan/
  2008report/Inventory_of_Projects_AR2008_01152010
  _final.pdf.
- A good *New York Times* article about fish farming in
  China: http://www.nytimes.com/2007/12/15/world/
  asia/15fish.html.

Mercury and Other Heavy Metals

- The EPA overview and links to additional information:
  http://www.epa.gov/waterscience/fishadvice/advice.html.
- An FDA advisory for pregnant, nursing women, and
  young mothers: http://www.fda.gov/Food/
  ResourcesForYou/Consumers/ucm110591.htm.
- *The New York Times* investigation of mercury in sushi:
  http://www.nytimes.com/2008/01/23/dining/23sushi
  .html.

PCBs and Dioxins

- For POPs in our fish: search *Environmental Health Perspectives* (http://ehsehplp03.niehs.nih.gov) for latest research.
- An overview of PCBs with special reference to children: http://healthychild.org/issues/chemical-pop/polychlorinated_biphenyls/.
- To calculate your risk: http://www.iatp.org/foodandhealth/fishcalculator/index.cfm.

Meat and Poultry

Microbes

- A readable and unsettling overview of *E. coli* O157:H7: Eric Schlosser, "Order the Fish," *Vanity Fair* (November 2004): 24. (Highlights the weakness of government and power of the meat industry.)
- An overview of ground beef safety issue: http://www.fsis.usda.gov/factsheets/ground_beef_and_food_safety/index.asp.

Parasites

- A USDA overview of main parasites: http://www.fsis.usda.gov/Fact_Sheets/Parasites_and_Foodborne_Illness/index.asp.
- A semitechnical overview, with pictures: http://www.aafp.org/afp/20040301/1161.html.

Hormones

- A critical view: http://www.sustainabletable.org/issues/hormones/.
- For those seriously concerned about links between hormones in food and early onset of puberty: D. Lindsey Berkson, *Hormone Deception* (Contemporary Books, 2000).

Antibiotics

- A quick introduction: http://www.who.int/mediacentre/factsheets/fs194/en/.
- A more technical discussion, including the economics: Silvia Secchi and Bruce A. Babcock, "Pearls Before Swine? Potential Trade-offs Between the Human and Animal Use of Antibiotics," *American Journal of Agricultural Economics*, http://www.jstor.org/pss/1245059.
- The National Research Council, Committee on Drug use in Food Animals, analysis of the issue (a little dated): *The Use of Drugs in Food Animals: Benefits and Risks* (National Academy Press, 1999).

Toxic Residues

- For a good insight into the arsenic-in-poultry issue—plus the other horrors of what our modern broilers are given in their feed: http://www.iatp.org/iatp/publications.cfm?accountID=421&refID=80529
- For an overview of those other toxic chemicals that could be in our meat (and dairy): http://www.agobservatory.org/library.cfm?refID=72846. This is a must-read for anyone with a young child.

BSE (Mad Cow Disease)

- A quick summary of the main risk issues: http://www.bseinfo.org/faq.Governmentregulations.aspx.
- The global situation and links to maps: http://www.oie.int/eng/info_ev/en_BSEHome.htm
- For the real story, and an excellent objective summary of the whole issue, see what Congress was told: http://fpc.state.gov/documents/organization/58240.pdf.
- Health Canada information on the issue and actions taken: http://www.hc-sc.gc.ca/fn-an/securit/animal/bse-esb/index-eng.php.
- The CFIA's answers to questions on BSE, and updates:

www.inspection.gc.ca/english/anima/heasan/disemala/
bseesb/bseesbindexe.shtml.

Avian Influenza

- A CDC summary of risks for humans: http://www.cdc
  .gov/flu/avian/.
- If traveling: http://www.who.int/csr/disease/avian
  _influenza/en/.

Swine Flu

- A general overview of the disease: http://www.cdc.gov/
  flu/swineflu/ and on: http://www.cdc.gov/flu/swineflu/
  key_facts.htm.

Nitrites

- If you want to forget this issue, the American Meat
  Institute will help: http://www.usdec.org/files/Deli/
  PDFs/3_US_Deli%20Meats.pdf.
- If you want to give up hot dogs forever: http://www
  .sustainabletable.org/features/articles/summerfun/
  hotdogdays.html.
- For a comprehensive and frightening look at the topic:
  Mike Adams, *Grocery Warning*, Truth Publishing, 2004.

Irradiation

- The basics: http://www.fns.usda.gov/cnd/Lunch/
  Downloadable/irrad.pdf.

Dairy

Bacteria

- For the CDC's view of risks in raw milk and dairy products:
  http://www.cdc.gov/healthypets/cheesespotlight/cheese
  _spotlight.htm.
- An overview of *Listeria* bacteria (in raw milk and other

foods): http://www.cdc.gov/nczved/dfbmd/disease
_listing/listeriosis_gi.html.

- To learn more about raw milk cheeses from an industry source: http://www.rawmilkcheese.org/index.htm.

Hormones

- Canada's review of the issue: http://www.parl.gc.ca /36/1/parlbus/commbus/senate/com-e/agri-e/rep-e/ repintermar99part1-e.htm.
- The industry's positive view of hormone use: http:// itisafact.org/media/510/facts%20about%20rbst%20june .pdf.
- For a balanced technical discussion of the issue: http:// www.consumersunion.org/pub/core_food_safety/002272 .html.

Antibiotics

- A brief but sound overview of antibiotic use by dairy industry: http://www.cvmbs.colostate.edu/ilm/proinfo/ cdn/2003/CDNmay03insert.pdf.

Molds

- A slightly technical review of research on the issue in dairy: http://jds.fass.org/cgi/reprint/64/12/2439.pdf.

Chemicals and Toxic Metals

- An overview of toxic chemicals, of special relevance to pregnant/nursing mothers: http://www.atsdr.cdc.gov/ tfacts35.html.
- If you are interested in the hypothesized link between autism and toxic metals in dairy: http://www.earthsave .org/news/vaccinesautism.htm.
- For an intellectually challenging report on risks of dioxins: http://www.ejnet.org/dioxin/nas2006.pdf.

Melamine
- The FDA summary of melamine situation in China and in U.S. food supply: http://www.fda.gov/NewsEvents/ PublicHealthFocus/ucm179005.htm.
- The WHO summary of the issue: http://www.who.int/ csr/media/faq/QAmelamine/en/index.html.

Eggs

Bacteria
- A clear if outdated discussion of the *Salmonella* issue: http://www.ers.usda.gov/publications/foodreview/ jan1997/jan97d.pdf.
- For more about the huge 2010 outbreak and recall: http:// www.fda.gov/Safety/Recalls/MajorProductRecalls/ ucm223522.htm.

Avian Influenza
- The CDC and WHO Web sites on bird flu also cover issues in eggs: http://www.cdc.gov/flu/avian/ and http:// www.who.int/csr/disease/avian_influenza/en/.

Antibiotic Residues
- For reassurance on the issue: Dan J. Donogue, "Antibiotic residues in poultry tissues and eggs: human health concerns?" Research Gate Scientific Network, www .researchgate.net/publication/10790413 or on NCBI at http://www.ncbi.nlm.nih.gov/pubmed/12710482.

Grains, Legumes, and Nuts

General Information about Grains, Legumes, and Nuts
- An overview of grains, including health benefits of some: http://www.wholegrainscouncil.org/whole-grains-101/ whole-grains-a-to-z/ or http://lpi.oregonstate.edu/ infocenter/foods/grains/.

- For a thoroughly clear explanation of the process of nitrogen fixation in legumes: http://aces.nmsu.edu/pubs/_a/a-129.pdf.
- To look up any nut, go to the Agriculture Marketing Resource Center at: http://www.agmrc.org/commodities_products/nuts/.

Microbes

- Detail on the 2008–2009 outbreaks of *Salmonella* in peanut butter and peanut products: http://www.cdc.gov/mmwr/preview/mmwrhtml/mm5804a4.htm.
- If tempted to think that tree nuts cannot become contaminated with bacteria: http://pubs.caes.uga.edu/caespubs/pubcd/C939/C939.htm.
- For information on the pistachio recall: http://www.accessdata.fda.gov/scripts/pistachiorecall/index.cfm.
- Comprehensive discussion of aflatoxin, with information on nuts: Hamed K. Abbas (ed.), *Aflatoxin and Food Safety* (CRC Press—Taylor and Francis, Boca Raton, Florida, 2005).
- A basic technical overview of aflatoxin: http://www.ansci.cornell.edu/plants/toxicagents/aflatoxin/aflatoxin.html.
- A Web site dedicated to aflatoxin, with special focus on peanuts: http://www.aflatoxin.info/introduction.asp.
- An overview of main mold toxins in corn (plus photos): http://www.ces.ncsu.edu/depts/pp/notes/Corn/corn001.htm.
- For a detailed account of the tortilla-related outbreak among schoolchildren: http://www.cdc.gov/mmwr/preview/mmwrhtml/00056731.htm, or the article by E. Steinburg, A. Henderson, A. Karpati., et al., "Mysterious Outbreaks of Gastrointestinal Illness Associated with Burritos Supplied Through School Lunch Programs," *Journal of Food Protection* 69 (2009).

- For a look at how the FDA tries to minimize the levels of mycotoxins in grains (although this is changing): http://www.fda.gov/downloads/Food/ucm073294.pdf.

Pesticides

- A technical overview of some common organochlorine contaminant groups and their risks: http://whale .wheelock.edu/bwcontaminants/contaminants.html.
- An official industry overview of PPO and other approaches nut sterilization: http://www.almondboard .com/FoodProfessionals/Documents/Pasteurization _Sheet%205.22.09.pdf.
- The EPA discussion of PPO at the time of reregistration, see http://edocket.access.gpo.gov/2005/E5-7625.htm.
- The manufacturer's arguments for PPO safety: http:// www.ars.usda.gov/is/np/mba/apr00/oxide.htm.

Heavy Metals

- The CDC summary of arsenic regulation: http://www .atsdr.cdc.gov/csem/arsenic/standards_regulations.html
- An overview of the arsenic issue in rice: http://www.pubmedcentral.nih.gov/articlerender .fcgi?artid=1892142.
- Or, for an easy-to-read article on the topic: http://www .newscientist.com/article/dn14592-superfood-rice-bran -contains-arsenic.html.
- For an overview of arsenic in *rice bran*: http://www.celsias .com/article/rice-bran-and-arsenic-unhealthy-health-food/.

Natural Toxins

- For reassurance on soy toxins from the industry: http:// www.soyfoods.org/health/faq#answer-1.
- A negative view of soy foods that at least mothers of infants should read: http://www.thyroid-info.com/ articles/soydangers.htm.

- To get more technical information on the animal studies done: http://humrep.oxfordjournals.org/cgi/content/full/17/7/1692.
- If you really want to get into the negative side of the topic, get hold of a copy of Kaayla T. Daniel, *The Whole Soy Story: the Dark Side of America's Favorite Health Food* (New Trend Publishing, 2009) or Dianne Gregg, *The Hidden Dangers of Soy* (Outskirts Press.com, 2008).

Herbs and Spices

General Information
- An interesting, but dated, overview of the spice market in the United States: http://www.ers.usda.gov/Publications/AIB709/.
- For the official definition and list of spices: http://www.accessdata.fda.gov/scripts/cdrh/cfdocs/cfcfr/CFRSearch.cfm?fr=501.22.
- The best source (unusually informative for an industry organization) on all information on spices: ASTA (The American Spice Trade Association) http://www.astaspice.org.

Bacteria
- An overview of the bacterial contamination issue in spices: http://www.astaspice.org/files/public/ASTA_Micro_Safety_White_Paper_Final.pdf2009.
- More technical discussion, with focus on actual outbreaks and *Salmonella*: http://cdc.gov/enterics/publications/381_vij.pdf.

Molds
- For research on which spices are likely to carry the most aflatoxin: http://www.ncbi.nlm.nih.gov/pubmed/7275911.

Toxic Dyes

- For an overview of Sudan dyes in spices, with links to regulation and other issues: http://www.separationsnow.com/coi/cda/detail.cda?id=16833&type=Feature&chId=4&page=1.

Acknowledgments

T<small>HIS</small> <small>BOOK</small> <small>HIJACKED</small> my life for longer than I expected. Graham, my husband, has made it clear that I had better start by thanking him. He has been remarkably good humored about all those evenings and weekends I spent with my computer, the vacations he had to take alone, and those many times when he wished I would spend less time talking about risks in food and more time cooking great meals and eating them. In addition, both he and my son, Douglas, have provided essential encouragement and good advice along the way. Then there are all those friends and colleagues who helped to shape this book, read early drafts, and provided feedback on key sections. Special thanks to Judith Beinstein Miller, professor emeritus, Oberlin College, and my close friend since graduate school in Philadelphia. Also to Marsha Echols, Professor at Howard University School of Law, Washington, D.C., and director of the World Food Law Institute. Without all of you, I would never have risen to the challenge, or survived to the last page.

To my agent, Amy Burkhardt, of Kimberley Cameron and Associates, and editor, Iris Bass. Nor can I leave out my publisher, Matthew Lore, who, in spite of all his time constraints, gave so much personal attention to this book. Thank you for becoming so involved in the topic, and for what you have done to improve the end product.

Finally, there are all those researchers around the world and staff at FDA, USDA, CFIA, and food industry associations, whom I have pestered with technical and policy questions. Thanks to those of you who patiently responded—and no thanks to those who did not.

Index

NOTE: Page numbers in **bold** indicate a glossary definition.

About the Author

HELI PERRETT, PHD, comes to the topic of food safety from several angles—her training and hands-on work experience in both the United States and Canada in public health microbiology; her personal background and international experience in food issues, farming, and public health; and her perspective as a sociologist. She has served as a senior technical adviser on the staff of the United Nations Development Agency in New York and as an adviser on health education and sanitation at the World Bank in Washington, D.C. In addition, she has consulted for many years for the International Fund for Agriculture Development, the Food and Agriculture Organization, the USDA, and other U.S. and global organizations. Dr. Perrett has lectured at the American University in Washington, D.C., and in Canada, Europe, and Latin America. She is author of numerous papers and articles (many published by the UN and the World Bank). She is a member of the American Public Health Association, of Slow Food USA (Berkeley Chapter), and of Community Supported Agriculture. She is also a food enthusiast who loves to cook and eat.